'This is a very valuable book for all interested in the study of traumatic stress at various levels of education. It is making traumatic stress research accessible for a large and global audience!'

Professor Miranda Olff, *Amsterdam UMC, Department of Psychiatry*

'*Traumatic Stress* is a small but mighty book that presents the most up-to-date information and research on PTSD and other stressor-related disorders clearly, concisely, comprehensively, and authoritatively. Seven tightly but accessibly-written chapters focus on diagnosis, prevalence, psychological theory, biological mechanisms, risk factors, the latest research on psychotherapy and pharmacotherapy, and, as a finale, a very unique and important chapter on the challenges of dissemination and implementation of evidence-based treatments. It is a superb resource for undergraduate, graduate, and post-graduate students as well as for non-specialist medical and mental health clinicians who want to learn about the science and practice of PTSD and related disorders.'

Matthew J. Friedman, MD, PhD, *Emeritus Professor,*
Geisel School of Medicine at Dartmouth

'This is everything you need to know about traumatic stress and posttraumatic stress disorder in an easy to read, highly digestible book. Perfect for new students or established clinicians who want a quick snapshot of where the evidence is at in terms of prevalence, treatment, biology, current psychological theories, and considerations for dissemination. I'll be recommending this to all my students!'

Professor Meaghan O'Donnell, *Head of Research, Centre for*
Posttraumatic Mental Health, The University of Melbourne

'This book is a great primer on all aspects of PTSD – from epidemiology, to risk factors and theoretical models for why and how PTSD develops, to treatment. The book is extremely comprehensive. It references a large amount of complicated research yet is written in a way that is both engaging and accessible. I would recommend this book to anyone who wants to come up to speed on what we know about PTSD and how to treat it.'

Sonya B. Norman, PhD, *Consultation Program Director at NCPTSD,*
National Center for PTSD, Professor, University of California
San Diego School of Medicine

'*Traumatic Stress* is the perfect book for anyone who wishes to achieve a concise, authoritative understanding of PTSD and other stressor-related disorders. The authors, Drs. Patricia Resick and Stefanie LoSavio, bring a rare combination of vast clinical and research experience, comprehensive knowledge of the field, and good writing to the task of telling us the essentials of what we need to know about traumatic stress without getting us lost in the weeds of peripheral details. Although the book will be most useful for those who know little about the topic and wish to get up to speed quickly, there is also valuable information in it for traumatic stress "experts" who could use a well-written overview and update of this complex field. In short, this is an excellent book that is a valuable contribution to the traumatic stress field.'

Dean G. Kilpatrick, PhD, *Distinguished University Professor,*
Medical University of South Carolina

'This slim volume packs a punch. *Traumatic Stress* is a compact, comprehensive primer on the basics of PTSD and other related trauma disorders. It distills the essential evidence base about trauma into clear, concise conceptual units that will resonate with a wide range of readers – from undergraduates to clinicians and researchers who need to update their competencies in traumatic stress studies. With the straight-forward, no-nonsense style that Resick is known for, she and her colleague Stefanie LoSavio simplify – without distorting – the essential knowledge that every trauma professional needs to know. This should be mandatory reading for all in the field who want to get a handle on the major science and theories shaping the field of traumatic stress.'

Elana Newman, PhD, *McFarlin Chair in Psychology,*
The University of Tulsa

Traumatic Stress

Traumatic Stress provides a well-written and accessible overview of traumatic stress studies. With its pioneering lead author, this book reviews the full range of clinical disorders that may result from extreme stress, with particular emphasis on posttraumatic stress disorder (PTSD). It synthesizes the current literature on traumatic stress, including psychological theories of stress and trauma; the biology of stress and trauma reactions; and the factors prior to, during, and after traumatic events that place people at particular risk for the development of psychological problems. It also covers the use of medication and a range of psychological treatments. Completely revamped with new case studies and research, the book gives important updates on biological research and therapy, as well as changes in diagnostic classifications.

The new edition will continue to be essential reading for undergraduate and postgraduate students, as well as busy professionals working in this field who want a concise update on disorders related to traumatic stress.

Patricia A. Resick, PhD, ABPP, is Professor Emeritus of Psychiatry and Behavioral Sciences at Duke University Medical School, has researched trauma for 50 years, and has received research and mentoring awards and lifetime achievement awards from the American Psychological Association (Trauma Division 56), International Society for Traumatic Stress Studies, and Association for Behavioral and Cognitive Therapies.

Stefanie T. LoSavio, PhD, ABPP, serves as Assistant Professor of Psychiatry and Behavioral Sciences at the University of Texas Health Science Center at San Antonio and Director of Research and Innovation at the STRONG STAR Training Initiative. Her research focuses on enhancing the effectiveness and reach of evidence-based treatments for PTSD.

Clinical Psychology: A Modular Course was designed to overcome the problems faced by the traditional textbook in conveying what psychological disorders are really like. All the books in the series, written by leading scholars and practitioners in the field, can be read as stand-alone texts, but they will also integrate with the other modules to form a comprehensive resource in clinical psychology. Students of psychology, medicine, nursing, and social work, as well as busy practitioners in many professions, often need an accessible but thorough introduction to how people experience anxiety, depression, addiction, or other disorders; how common they are; and who is most likely to suffer from them, as well as up-to-date research evidence on the causes and available treatments. The series will appeal to those who want to go deeper into the subject than the traditional textbook will allow, and base their examination answers, research, projects, assignments, or practical decisions on a clearer and more rounded appreciation of the clinical and research evidence.

Chris R. Brewin

For a full list of titles in the series, please visit the Routledge website at: https://www.routledge.com/Clinical-Psychology-A-Modular-Course/book-series/SE0543

Traumatic Stress

Second Edition

Patricia A. Resick and Stefanie T. LoSavio

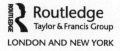

Routledge
Taylor & Francis Group

LONDON AND NEW YORK

Designed cover image: © Getty Images

Second edition published 2025
by Routledge
4 Park Square, Milton Park, Abingdon, Oxon, OX14 4RN

and by Routledge
605 Third Avenue, New York, NY 10158

Routledge is an imprint of the Taylor & Francis Group, an informa business

© 2025 Patricia A. Resick and Stefanie T. LoSavio

First edition published by Routledge 2001

British Library Cataloguing-in-Publication Data
A catalogue record for this book is available from the British Library

ISBN: 978-0-367-33090-3 (hbk)
ISBN: 978-0-367-33088-0 (pbk)
ISBN: 978-0-429-31793-4 (ebk)

DOI: 10.4324/9780429317934

Typeset in Times New Roman
by codeMantra

Contents

Acknowledgments

First, we would like to thank the hundreds of researchers who have dedicated their lives to understanding all aspects of traumatic stress. This book summarizes a large literature, and there is more research than could possibly be included in this small volume. However, we recognize all the efforts that have brought the field where it is today. We would like to thank Chris Brewin, the series editor, for his generous patience and helpful suggestions. We also thank Grace McDonnell and Sarah Hafeez of Taylor & Francis for their assistance. Finally, we would like to thank our husbands for their constant support of our work, including the long hours spent preparing this book.

Preface

Normally when someone writes or edits an academic book, they revise it every five years or so. The book I wrote, *Stress and Trauma*, was originally published in 2001. I am a bit delayed on the second edition. I am sorry for that. In 2003 I moved to Boston to become the Director of the Women's Health Science Division (WHSD) of the National Center for PTSD. I had to pivot from research and clinical work with women who had been sexually or physically victimized to growing the WHSD and starting the dissemination of cognitive processing therapy throughout the Department of Veterans Affairs. Then, in 2013, I moved to a research position at Duke University Medical Center. I was working with large collaboratives on treatment research with active duty military service members. Finally, I started on a retirement track, put my head up, and thought I could start working on the second edition of the textbook. However, I soon realized that the field had changed so much that this would not be a revision but a complete rewrite. In fact, there is no longer room to discuss general information on stress. There are several diagnoses to cover in this new edition: PTSD, acute stress disorder, adjustment disorder, and prolonged grief disorder.

Because this volume has changed so much due to the explosion of research on all of the topics of this book over the past two decades, I asked a colleague, Stefanie LoSavio, PhD, ABPP, to co-author this book with me. This book is probably 90% new material. There are seven chapters: diagnoses, prevalence, theory, biology, risk factors, treatment, and dissemination. The lion's share of research has been conducted with PTSD, but other diagnoses will be covered when there is available research. The new name of the book is *Traumatic Stress*.

This book is aimed at undergraduates as part of a trauma course or an abnormal psychology course or for graduate students or professionals who want a crash course in traumatic stress. We intentionally reviewed a large amount of sometimes complicated research and then summarized it into more digestible concepts and conclusions. We hope you find this book to be a good resource for you to learn about traumatic stress.

Patricia A. Resick, PhD, ABPP

1

Introduction and Classifying Reactions to Traumatic Stress

Consider the following scenarios:

You are driving down a busy highway on a rainy day when your front tire has a blowout. Your first response is one of action, trying to pull the car over to the side of the road while avoiding a collision with other cars. You can't control the car and hit a car that was also pulling over. A child in the back seat was severely injured, as were you. You are haunted by thoughts of how you could have reacted differently and prevented the crash. Thoughts of it intrude every time you have to drive on a rainy day. You are jumpy whenever driving, and if someone slams on their brakes ahead of you, you have a startle response and start hyperventilating so badly that sometimes you must pull over just to calm yourself down.

You have been on deployment for 9 months and have seen very little action. A few days before you are to return home, your best buddy is on patrol with you. Without warning, you find yourself under fire. Your friend is killed, and you receive a wound in the arm. You are shipped to a hospital in Germany and then directly back to your base. You try not to think or talk about the incident and were not able to go to your friend's funeral in California. After being discharged from the military, you return to your hometown. You have nightmares and can't decide whether to go back to school or get a job, and

DOI: 10.4324/9780429317934-1

you avoid people, thinking about the traumatic event, or talking to anyone about your time in the service. Secretly you blame yourself for the death of your friend and feel guilt that you should have prevented it.

You are peacefully asleep in your bed when suddenly you are awakened by a voice that says, "I have a knife, so don't make any noise." You wonder if you are having a nightmare, but as you awaken more fully, you feel the point of the knife at your throat. You begin to panic as you experience complete terror. You feel frozen both mentally and physically.

You were physically and emotionally abused as a child, and a few years after high school you meet a man who treats you well and is kind. However, six months after marrying him, you have a fight over whether to have a baby right away. He hits you across the face. He is immediately apologetic and says it will never happen again. Six months later, while you are pregnant and exhausted, you tell him that you don't want to have sex. He hits you again, this time with his fist, and you have a black eye the next day.

All of these are examples of traumatic stress. Stressors may be positive (a promotion at work, a wedding) as well as negative. The stress response is a combination of physical reactions, thoughts (cognitions), emotions, and behaviors. The examples above represent *traumatic stress*, a more severe type of stressor that can result in several types of psychological disorders. In the first example, the car accident, there were injuries to self and a child. In the second example, a combat ambush, the service member is injured, and a good friend is killed. The third example is a sudden, unexpected, life-threatening assault. The last example is one of multiple traumas, including childhood maltreatment and adult intimate partner violence.

The focus of this book will be on traumatic stressors, which are events beyond daily hassles; beyond normal developmental life challenges; and beyond more stressful and challenging circumstances such as divorce, losing a job, illness, or financial problems. This book will focus on events that involve physical threats to safety, like life-threatening events, serious physical harm, or sexual violation, which may occur to a person or their significant others and result in a range of symptoms.

For some people, traumatic stressors may result in psychological disorders. This chapter will focus on the various psychological disorders that may result from traumatic stress. Chapter 2 will examine the prevalence of these most serious types of stressors and related psychological disorders. The remaining chapters will focus on theories of traumatic stress response, the biology of the traumatic stress response, variables that affect symptoms and recovery, treatment, and dissemination. The field of traumatic stress has exploded over the past several decades, a topic of study that did not exist at all before 1980 when the diagnosis of posttraumatic stress disorder

(PTSD) was first introduced. The purpose of this book is to provide an overview of the various topics that have received the most attention by researchers while condensing what is sometimes very technical into a concise and readable summary.

Traumatic Stress Recovery Patterns

Although a range of symptoms are common after a traumatic event, for some, recovery does not occur or the symptoms grow worse over time. When the psychological symptoms persist following a traumatic stressor and cluster into particular patterns, it is time to consider whether these reactions meet criteria for a psychopathological condition. The remainder of this section will describe various psychological disorders that are frequently observed following trauma.

Although almost any disorder might follow in the wake of a traumatic experience, there are specific disorders that are more frequent and will be focused on in this chapter. One thing to keep in mind is that most people recover from even very serious traumatic events and do not develop diagnosable disorders or, if diagnosed for a period, may still recover on their own. For example, PTSD is diagnosed after one month, but there is research showing that people continue to recover from their initial symptoms after that point in time. One of the myths that exists in the media and in the community is that if you have PTSD, you cannot recover from it. In a study that examined completed rapes prospectively starting at one-week post-rape, almost all the women met criteria for PTSD (except for the time criterion) at that point, but by three months post-rape, 48% had PTSD and the other 52% had recovered (Rothbaum et al., 1992).

Norris and Kaniasty (1994) examined the recovery of violent crime victims and property crime victims, comparing them with nonvictims at three time periods: 3, 9, and 15 months post-crime. They assessed a range of emotional reactions and found that while the crime victims showed substantial improvement between three and nine months post-crime, there was no improvement after that. As expected, the violent crime victims reported more distress than the property crime victims, who reported more distress than the nonvictims at each assessment point.

More recently, Monson et al. (2021) examined trauma victims within six months of their most recent traumatic event and then four times over the following year. About 53% were initially diagnosed with PTSD (similar to the previous studies) following a range of interpersonal or accidental traumatic events. By the final assessment, only 16% still had PTSD.

There have been a handful of studies that have prospectively examined reactions to serious motor vehicle accidents or natural disasters (e.g., Blanchard et al., 1996; Green et al., 1992; Mayou et al., 1993; McFarlane, 1988). Generally, these studies also have found that people continued to recover over the course of a year. Typically, symptoms are most severe at the earliest time point, and the rates of PTSD decrease over time. However, several studies have found that a small percentage of people have a delayed onset of PTSD (typically 3–5%). In these cases, those with a delayed onset of full diagnosis did not start with no symptoms; they had a partial diagnosis and then worsened over time until they met criteria for diagnosis. Blanchard et al. (1996) tracked 132 victims of motor vehicle accidents for 18 months and found that of the 48 individuals (36%) who met criteria for PTSD at one to four months post-accident, half had improved at least somewhat by six months post-accident, and two-thirds by the one-year follow-up. There was no significant improvement from 1 year to 18 months post-accident. When recovery stalls out and symptoms persist, a diagnosis and perhaps treatment are needed.

Posttraumatic Stress Disorder

DSM-5 and ICD-11

Until the International Classification of Diseases, 11th Edition (ICD-11; World Health Organization, 2019) was produced (and took effect in 2022), the diagnoses regarding traumatic stress were fairly parallel to the Diagnostic and Statistical Manual of Mental Disorders, Fifth Edition (DSM-5; American Psychiatric Association, 2013). Both the DSM-5 in 2013 and the ICD-11 in 2019 moved PTSD and related disorders out of the anxiety disorders category and into their own classification category, Trauma- and Stressor-Related Disorders (DSM-5) and Disorders Specifically Associated with Stress (ICD-11). This was an important change because when listed as an anxiety disorder, clinicians and researchers tended to overlook people whose primary emotion was anger, shame, or guilt and who might not experience fear and anxiety as the predominant emotion.

When the DSM-5 was produced in 2013, the individual items were examined with a default toward keeping items unless there was sufficient research to justify removing them. By the same token, items and categories could only be added if there was sufficient research to support it. Because individual items had not been examined during the revisions of the DSM-III, there was an abundance of evidence to support some new items and eventually a new criterion. The ICD-11 took a different direction with a more stripped-down simple PTSD category and a diagnosis of complex PTSD (CPTSD), which the DSM-IV and DSM-5 committees (e.g., Friedman et al., 2011) had examined and rejected. Therefore, there were many changes to the diagnosis of PTSD and some changes to acute stress disorder (ASD) and adjustment disorder in the DSM-5. The DSM-5 and ICD-11 will be described separately.

DSM-5 Criteria

In the DSM-5, the stressor criterion was rewritten to reflect the seriousness of the event and its impact on the person at the time of the event. Under the DSM-III-R (American Psychological Association, 1987), the description of the stressor was that the event was outside the normal range of events. This statement, of course, does not reflect the reality of the prevalence of traumatic events in people's lives. Although they are not "normal" events, if most of the population has experienced at least one major traumatic event in their lives, and some people have experienced many such events, the statement is not an accurate guideline for making the diagnosis.

According to the DSM-5, there are eight criteria that must be met before a diagnosis of PTSD can be made (see Box 1.1). The first criterion is the stressor Criterion A. A person has to have experienced or witnessed actual or threatened death, serious injury, or sexual violence; learned about such a traumatic event happening to a loved one; or experienced repeated or extreme exposure to aversive details of such a traumatic event(s), typically through work (e.g., first responders or military collecting human remains; police officers repeatedly exposed to details of child abuse). This definition allows a diagnosis not just for the direct victims themselves but also for affected family members such as the families of homicide victims or those who are not directly victimized such as those who work in the aftermath of violence or disaster. It also allows for a diagnosis in cases where no life threat is made but more explicitly through sexual violence such as rape or child sexual abuse.

BOX 1.1 Diagnostic Criteria for Posttraumatic Stress Disorder in DSM-5 (309.81)

Reprinted with permission from Diagnostic and Statistical Manual of Mental Disorders, Fifth Edition (Copyright © 2013). American Psychiatric Association. All Rights Reserved.

Note: The following criteria apply to adults, adolescents, and children older than 6 years.

A. Exposure to actual or threatened death, serious injury, or sexual violence in one (or more) of the following ways:

1. Directly experiencing the traumatic event(s).
2. Witnessing, in person, the event(s) as it occurred to others.

3. Learning that the traumatic event(s) occurred to a close family member or close friend. **Note:** In cases of actual or threatened death of a family member or friend, the event(s) must have been violent or accidental.
4. Experiencing repeated or extreme exposure to aversive details of the traumatic event(s) (e.g., first responders collecting human remains; police officers repeatedly exposed to details of child abuse).
Note: This does not apply to exposure through electronic media, television, movies, or pictures, unless this exposure is work related.

B. Presence of one (or more) of the following intrusion symptoms associated with the traumatic event(s), beginning after the traumatic event(s) occurred:

1. Recurrent, involuntary, and intrusive distressing memories of the traumatic event(s).
Note: In children older than 6 years, repetitive play may occur in which themes or aspects of the traumatic event(s) are expressed.
2. Recurrent distressing dreams in which the content and/or affect of the dream are related to the traumatic event(s).
Note: In children, there may be frightening dreams without recognizable content.
3. Dissociative reactions (e.g., flashbacks) in which the individual feels or acts as if the traumatic event(s) were recurring. (Such reactions may occur on a continuum, with the most extreme expression being a complete loss of awareness of present surroundings.)
Note: In children, trauma-specific reenactment may occur in play.
4. Intense or prolonged psychological distress at exposure to internal or external cues that symbolize or resemble an aspect of the traumatic event(s).
5. Marked physiological reactions to internal or external cues that symbolize or resemble an aspect of the traumatic event(s).

C. Persistent avoidance of stimuli associated with the traumatic event(s), beginning after the traumatic event(s) occurred, as evidenced by one or both of the following:

1. Avoidance of or efforts to avoid distressing memories, thoughts, or feelings about or closely associated with the traumatic event(s).
2. Avoidance of or efforts to avoid external reminders (people, places, conversations, activities, objects, situations) that arouse distressing

memories, thoughts, or feelings about or closely associated with the traumatic event(s).

D. Negative alterations in cognitions and mood associated with the traumatic event(s), beginning or worsening after the traumatic event(s) occurred, as evidenced by two (or more) of the following:

1. Inability to remember an important aspect of the traumatic event(s) (typically due to dissociative amnesia, and not to other factors such as head injury, alcohol, or drugs).
2. Persistent and exaggerated negative beliefs or expectations about one-self, others, or the world (e.g., "I am bad", "No one can be trusted", "The world is completely dangerous", "My whole nervous system is permanently ruined").
3. Persistent, distorted cognitions about the cause or consequences of the traumatic event(s) that lead the individual to blame himself/herself or others.
4. Persistent negative emotional state (e.g., fear, horror, anger, guilt, or shame).
5. Markedly diminished interest or participation in significant activities.
6. Feelings of detachment or estrangement from others.
7. Persistent inability to experience positive emotions (e.g., inability to experience happiness, satisfaction, or loving feelings).

E. Marked alterations in arousal and reactivity associated with the traumatic event(s), beginning or worsening after the traumatic event(s) occurred, as evidenced by two (or more) of the following:

1. Irritable behavior and angry outbursts (with little or no provocation), typically expressed as verbal or physical aggression toward people or objects.
2. Reckless or self-destructive behavior.
3. Hypervigilance.
4. Exaggerated startle response.
5. Problems with concentration.
6. Sleep disturbance (e.g., difficulty falling or staying asleep or restless sleep).

F. Duration of the disturbance (Criteria B, C, D and E) is more than 1 month.

G. The disturbance causes clinically significant distress or impairment in social, occupational, or other important areas of functioning.
H. The disturbance is not attributable to the physiological effects of a substance (e.g., medication, alcohol) or another medical condition.

Specify whether:

With dissociative symptoms: The individual's symptoms meet the criteria for posttraumatic stress disorder, and in addition, in response to the stressor, the individual experiences persistent or recurrent symptoms of either of the following:

1. **Depersonalization:** Persistent or recurrent experiences of feeling detached from, and as if one were an outside observer of, one's mental processes or body (e.g., feeling as though one were in a dream; feeling a sense of unreality of self or body or of time moving slowly).
2. **Derealization:** Persistent or recurrent experiences of unreality of surroundings (e.g., the world around the individual is experienced as unreal, dreamlike, distant, or distorted).
   Note: To use this subtype, the dissociative symptoms must not be attributable to the physiological effects of a substance (e.g., blackouts, behavior during alcohol intoxication) or another medical condition (e.g., complex partial seizures).

Specify if:

With delayed expression: If the full diagnostic criteria are not met until at least 6 months after the event (although the onset and expression of some symptoms may be immediate).

Under the age of 6 years, Criterion A includes learning that the traumatic event occurred to a parent or caregiving figure. Children often develop PTSD symptoms following terrorist attacks, even when they experience the attack indirectly through media exposure.

The second criterion, Criterion B, reflects intrusion symptoms. A person can meet this criterion if they have recurrent, unwanted, and distressing recollections of the traumatic event. The recollections may take the form of intrusive images, flashbacks, nightmares, or strong emotional or physical reactions when the person encounters reminders of the event. The person only needs one type of reexperiencing symptom to meet the criterion as long as this is recurrent and distressing. The random thought or occasional dream would not be of sufficient severity to be considered a problem. Intentional rumination about the trauma (e.g., "What if I had done this instead of that?") also does not count as an intrusive symptom. Criterion B is the same for children (one of the intrusive symptoms) except that spontaneous and intrusive memories may not necessarily appear distressing and may be expressed as play reenactment. The child can have dissociative episodes that can occur on a continuum and can occur during play. It may not be possible to determine if the content in dreams is related to the traumatic event.

Avoidance symptoms comprise the third criterion (Criterion C). This criterion has been changed the most from DSM-IV to DSM-5. In DSM-IV, people must have experienced three of seven types of avoidance. Many factor analysis studies found that the items did not hang together as a single type of avoidance. They usually fell into effortful avoidance or numbing but also factored into a dysphoria (depressive symptoms) factor. The DSM-5 Criterion C has been reduced to two items: avoidance of internal memories or avoidance of external reminders. However, there are probably thousands of ways in which someone could achieve internal or external avoidance (e.g., keeping extremely busy, avoiding places or people who are reminders, substance use).

Symptoms of negative alterations in cognition and mood are represented in Criterion D. This criterion was added to the DSM-5 because of so much research on both cognitions like distorted blame of self or others for the cause of the traumatic event and the effects beyond fear such as shame, guilt, or anger. One must experience at least two of these symptoms.

Criterion E includes pervasive arousal that is reflected by difficulties in concentration, hypervigilance, irritability, and problems falling and staying asleep. Also included are exaggerated startle responses to stimuli. There is evidence that many of those with PTSD not only have pronounced startle reactions, but they do not appear to habituate to repeated presentations of stimuli as do people without PTSD. A new addition to this criterion, which is now called "arousal and reactivity", is irritable behavior or angry outbursts (as differentiated from angry mood). Another new addition is reckless or self-destructive behavior (e.g., speeding, motorcycle riding without a helmet, cutting). These two symptoms help bridge the gap with CPTSD along with the Criterion D symptoms and may result from attempts to modulate affect.

Criterion F for diagnosis is that the B, C, D, and E symptoms persist for at least a month. In other words, someone would not meet the criteria for PTSD if they had avoidance symptoms at one period of time and nightmares and flashbacks at another or if the symptoms lasted just a week or two. The symptoms must co-occur together for at least one month. The last criterion is that this combination of symptoms causes significant distress for the person or causes impairment in the person's social or occupational functioning. This last criterion, present for all disorders, specifies that a diagnosis of psychopathology should not be made if the symptoms are mild or do not really interfere with a person's life. Diagnosis of psychological disorders should not be made frivolously and should indicate the need for treatment. Mild or occasional symptoms fall within the range of normal reactions to stressful events.

Dissociative subtype of PTSD: Following a series of studies from different fields such as epidemiology (Wolf et al., 2012, 2017), psychophysiology (Griffin et al., 1997), brain imaging (Lanius and colleagues, 2002, 2010, 2012), and treatment (Resick et al., 2012), a dissociative subtype was added to the DSM-5. In all cases, there was a small but significant subset of PTSD patients who reacted differently with high levels of dissociation. The two symptoms of the dissociative subtype are derealization (feeling unreal or detached from the world) and/or depersonalization (feeling that one's body is detached from the self).

ICD-11 Criteria

PTSD has been separated out from CPTSD in the ICD-11 (World Health Organization, 2018). From the perspective of user ease, the ICD-11 PTSD diagnosis has no categories and a minimal number of symptoms that are unique to PTSD. The other goal of revisions to the ICD-11 was to reduce comorbid diagnoses by eliminating symptoms that overlap with other disorders. Another purpose of having minimal symptoms in the PTSD diagnosis is for ease of administration and diagnosis throughout the world (Brewin et al., 2017). The difference between the ICD-11 and DSM-5 is that the ICD-11 focuses on identifying the minimal number of symptoms to identify the disorder, whereas the DSM-5 describes the most common symptoms of PTSD.

The symptoms of ICD-11 PTSD are reduced to three elements such that the person must have one from each category (compared to six symptoms needed in the DSM-5): (1) reexperiencing the trauma in the present, dissociative flashbacks, or nightmares; (2) avoidance of external reminders or avoidance of thoughts; and (3) persistent sense of threat indicated by hypervigilance or exaggerated startle response. There is also an impairment criterion, but there is no minimum time criterion like the DSM-5, just that the symptoms should last at least a few weeks. The trauma criterion is defined as an extremely threatening or horrific event or series of events. According to Brewin et al. (2017), an essential feature of the reexperiencing symptoms is that they are not just remembered but are experienced as if they are occurring again in the here and now. Both avoidance and a heightened sense of threat are essential features of the ICD-11. This is clearly different from the DSM-5, which allows for PTSD diagnosis with a deep sense of guilt, shame, or anger, not just fear. The ICD-11 does not have a dissociative subtype, but it is one of the core variations of PTSD.

The other dramatic change in the ICD-11 was the inclusion of a diagnosis of CPTSD. Although considered and rejected twice for the DSM, due to lack of evidence that it was different than severe PTSD, the authors of the ICD decided that there was enough evidence to include a separate disorder, CPTSD. The ICD-10 also had a disorder that preceded CPTSD, Enduring Personality Change After Catastrophic Experience. However, unlike the new PTSD criteria with seven items and three clusters of symptoms, namely, reexperiencing, avoidance, and arousal/sense of threat (Brewin et al., 2017), CPTSD has six clusters including the three from PTSD and three others regarding disturbances in self-organization (DSO): affect dysregulation, negative self-concept, and difficulties in relationships. They have specified that CPTSD does not require a personality change, which would be difficult to justify if the abuse started very early in life, but that these symptom clusters are pervasive and ongoing. It is assumed that CPTSD results most often from early and ongoing abuse but could also result from any repeated traumas from which escape is not possible such as domestic violence, torture, or war imprisonment.

Acute Stress Disorder

Sylvia was alone in her second-story apartment when the earthquake struck. She felt the floor beneath her give way, and she had nothing to grab onto as furniture, objects, and walls fell around her. An hour later, emergency workers found her walking in a daze with her dead cat in her arms. She had cuts and bruises but did not appear to be in pain, and she did not respond when the emergency workers asked her if anyone else was inside her apartment. A week later, she had strong panic attacks whenever there were aftershocks or if she heard a loud truck rumbling. She had nightmares about falling and had no memory of the hour after the earthquake, how she got outside, or of finding her cat. She described herself as numb and "just going through the motions".

DSM-5 Criteria

ASD was introduced with the DSM-IV following research findings that those people who dissociate more during or immediately after a traumatic stressor (peritraumatic dissociation) are more likely to develop chronic PTSD (Spiegel et al., 1996). The introduction of this disorder allowed for a diagnosis in the first month after an event without including those who would recover naturally during that interval. Under the DSM-IV, ASD required the same Criterion A definition of a traumatic stressor as PTSD (see earlier), but Criterion B required three or more dissociative symptoms experienced during or after the event. The five symptoms that qualified for this criterion were (1) numbing or detachment, (2) reduced awareness of surroundings (being in a daze), (3) derealization, (4) depersonalization, or (5) dissociative amnesia (inability to recall an important aspect of the trauma). Derealization is a sense of unreality or that the situation is not real. The person who says repeatedly, "I couldn't believe it was really happening" or "It felt like a dream" or "Everything seemed distorted and unreal" is expressing a sense of derealization. Depersonalization is more a sense that the person themselves is not real. The person may experience the traumatic event as if they are floating above their body or from somewhere else outside their body.

In addition to the dissociative symptoms, the affected person must have experienced symptoms from each of the PTSD symptom clusters. However, the complete criteria for PTSD did not need to be met. Only one symptom from each criterion was required. Criterion C is that the person persistently reexperiences the event through recurrent images, thoughts, dreams, illusions, flashbacks, or distress upon exposure to reminders of the traumatic event. Criterion D includes marked avoidance of reminders or thoughts of the event. Criterion E is symptoms of anxiety or increased physiological arousal such as difficulties with sleep, irritability, poor concentration, hypervigilance, exaggerated startle response, or motor restlessness.

As in the current DSM-5, the DSM-IV criteria for ASD indicated that the symptoms must cause clinically significant distress or impairment in social or work functioning or impair the person from pursuing some necessary task such as obtaining assistance or mobilizing social support (Criterion F). The symptoms must last a minimum of two days (three in DSM-5) and a maximum of four weeks and must occur within four weeks of the event (Criterion G). The symptoms also must not be caused by some substance such as drugs or medication or a medical condition (Criterion H).

The inclusion of ASD in the DSM-IV had been controversial because so little research had been conducted to warrant this new diagnostic category and because of the inclusion of so many dissociation items. Some psychiatrists and psychologists argued that such an addition to the diagnostic system was premature given the lack of evidence that ASD symptoms represent a unique syndrome, that it does not predict later PTSD diagnosis better than a simple examination of early PTSD symptoms, or that initial reactions following trauma represent psychopathology at all. However, the addition of ASD to the DSM-IV spurred research regarding early detection and predictors of PTSD. Although not studied as much as PTSD, ASD has now had some research attention, and the criteria for the DSM-5 have changed.

ASD had two purposes: to serve as a diagnosis so that people who were immediately suffering could reach out for treatment if a diagnosis were needed, and as a possible predictor for who would develop PTSD to triage people most likely to need follow-up, especially in cases where resources are limited. Unfortunately, the latter purpose was not met, perhaps because the dissociative symptoms were too restrictive

(Bryant et al., 2011). The DSM-IV required three different types of dissociative symptoms and then at least one type of intrusion, arousal, and avoidance.

Although it did provide a diagnosis for early symptoms, ASD did not prove to be a good predictor of who would develop PTSD (Bryant, 2011). In an examination of 22 studies, Bryant found mixed results on whether ASD predicted later PTSD, but, importantly, many who would develop chronic PTSD did not begin with ASD symptoms (Bryant et al., 2008). For this reason, the DSM-5 did not emphasize the predictive value of ASD but its usefulness as an early diagnostic disorder for receiving treatment when a diagnosis is needed.

The DSM-5 diagnostic criteria decreased the emphasis on dissociation and do not require particular symptoms from different categories, but at least nine symptoms across types of posttrauma symptoms (see Box 1.2).

BOX 1.2 Diagnostic Criteria for Acute Stress Disorder in DSM-5 (308.3)

Reprinted with permission from Diagnostic and Statistical Manual of Mental Disorders, Fifth Edition, (Copyright © 2013). American Psychiatric Association. All Rights Reserved.

A. Exposure to actual or threatened death, serious injury, or sexual violence in one (or more) of the following ways:

1. Directly experiencing the traumatic event(s).
2. Witnessing, in person, the event(s) as it occurred to others.
3. Learning that the traumatic event(s) occurred to a close family member or close friend. **Note.** In cases of actual or threatened death of a family member or friend, the event(s) must have been violent or accidental.
4. Experiencing repeated or extreme exposure to aversive details of the traumatic event(s) (e.g., first responders collecting human remains; police officers repeatedly exposed to details of child abuse).
   Note: This does not apply to exposure through electronic media, television, movies, or pictures, unless this exposure is work related.

B. Presence of nine (or more) of the following symptoms from any of the five categories of intrusion, negative mood, dissociation, avoidance, and arousal, beginning or worsening after the traumatic event(s) occurred.
Intrusion Symptoms

1. Recurrent, involuntary, and intrusive distressing memories of the traumatic event(s).
    Note: In children, repetitive play may occur in which the themes or aspects of the traumatic event(s) are expressed.
2. Recurrent distressing dreams in which the content and/or affect of the dream are related to the event(s).
    Note: In children, there may be frightening dreams without recognizable content.
3. Dissociative reactions (e.g., flashbacks) in which the individual feels or acts as if the traumatic event(s) were recurring. (Such reactions may occur on a continuum, with the most extreme expression being a complete loss of awareness of present surroundings.)
    Note: In children, trauma-specific reenactment may occur in play.
4. Intense or prolonged psychological distress or marked physiological reactions in response to internal or external cues that symbolize or resemble an aspect of the traumatic event(s).

Negative Mood

5. Persistent inability to experience positive emotions (e.g., inability to experience happiness, satisfaction, or loving feelings).

Dissociative Symptoms

6. An altered sense of the reality of one's surroundings or oneself (e.g., seeing oneself from another's perspective, being in a daze, time slowing).
7. Inability to remember an important aspect of the traumatic event(s) (typically due to dissociative amnesia and not to other factors such as head injury, alcohol, or drugs).

Avoidance Symptoms

8. Efforts to avoid distressing memories, thoughts, or feelings about or closely associated with the traumatic event(s).
9. Efforts to avoid external reminders (people, places, conversations, activities, objects, situations) that arouse distressing memories, thoughts, or feelings about or closely associated with the traumatic event(s).

Arousal Symptoms

10. Sleep disturbance (e.g., difficulty falling or staying asleep, restless sleep)

11. Irritable behavior and angry outbursts (with little or no provocation), typically expressed as verbal or physical aggression toward people or objects
12. Hypervigilance
13. Problems with concentration
14. Exaggerated startle response

C. Duration of the disturbance (symptoms in Criterion B) is three days to one month after trauma exposure.
   Note: Symptoms typically begin immediately after the trauma, but persistence for at least three days and up to a month is needed to meet disorder criteria.

D. The disturbance causes clinically significant distress or impairment in social, occupational, or other important areas of functioning.

E. The disturbance is not attributable to the physiological effects of a substance (e.g., medication or alcohol) or another medical condition (e.g., mild traumatic brain injury) and is not better explained by brief psychotic disorder.

ICD-11 Criteria

The ICD takes a different approach to ASD compared to the DSM. Because it was not a good predictor of the development of PTSD and PTSD can be diagnosed immediately after the trauma in ICD-11, there is no ICD-11 ASD diagnosis but instead acute stress reaction, a normal reaction to trauma that begins to subside very quickly after trauma, often within a week after the termination of the traumatic stressor.

Adjustment Disorder

Marcus, aged 9, returned home from school one day to find his mother crying. She informed him that his father had left and she didn't know how they would get money to live. For the first few days, he didn't react very much, but as it became clear to him that his father wasn't returning, he began to react in a variety of ways. Every time his mother needed to leave him with his grandmother, Marcus became tearful and clingy. This separation fear evolved into temper tantrums within a few weeks as his mother found a job that required her to be gone until 5:30 in the evening. He cried easily, lost his temper frequently, and had trouble getting along with his friends. His grades at school dropped. Marcus' mother sought counseling, and Marcus met with a school psychologist on a number of occasions. Within four or five months, Marcus began to adapt to the new situation, his reactions abated, and his behavior improved. His mother had similar responses of anxiety and depression that improved over a period of months as she was able to obtain a job and settle into a new pattern of life with her son.

BOX 1.3   Diagnostic Criteria for Adjustment Disorder in DSM-5 (309)

Reprinted with permission from Diagnostic and Statistical Manual of Mental Disorders, Fifth Edition, (Copyright © 2013). American Psychiatric Association. All Rights Reserved.

A. The development of emotional or behavioral symptoms in response to an identifiable stressor(s) occurring within 3 months of the onset of the stressor(s).
B. These symptoms or behaviors are clinically significant, as evidenced by one or both of the following:

   1. Marked distress that is out of proportion to the severity or intensity of the stressor, taking into account the external context and the cultural factors that might influence symptom severity and presentation.
   2. Significant impairment in social, occupational, or other important areas of functioning.

C. The stress-related disturbance does not meet the criteria for another mental disorder and is not merely an exacerbation of a preexisting mental disorder.
D. The symptoms do not represent normal bereavement.
E. Once the stressor or its consequences have terminated, the symptoms do not persist for more than an additional 6 months.

Specify whether:
   309.0 (F43.21) With depressed mood: Low mood, tearfulness, or feelings of hopelessness are predominant.
   309.24 (F43.22) With anxiety: Nervousness, worry, jitteriness, or separation anxiety is predominant.
   309.28 (F43.23) With mixed anxiety and depressed mood: A combination of depression and anxiety is predominant.

309.3 (F43.24) With disturbance of conduct: Disturbance of conduct is predominant.

309.4 (F43.25) With mixed disturbance of emotions and conduct: Both emotional symptoms (e.g., depression, anxiety) and a disturbance of conduct are predominant.

309.9 (F43.20) Unspecified: For maladaptive reactions that are not classifiable as one of the specific subtypes of adjustment disorder.

Specify if:
   Acute: if the disturbance lasts less than 6 months
   Persistent (chronic): if the disturbance lasts for 6 months or longer

DSM-5 Criteria

In the DSM-5, adjustment disorder was moved into the Trauma- and Stressor-Related Disorders chapter, which gave it more legitimacy. Like ASD, adjustment disorder is a catch-all classification so that someone who does not meet criteria for other disorders may have a diagnosis that will allow reimbursable therapy. The major difference is that ASD requires a traumatic stressor and a specific number of PTSD-type symptoms, while adjustment disorder follows an identifiable life event such as divorce or work problems, or even a stressful developmental event like leaving home for the first time, becoming a parent, or retirement. However, while these events are often stressful, the reaction would be excessive from what most other people experience. Adjustment disorder can be used in the case of bereavement if the reactions are excessive in intensity, quality, or persistence. However, a new diagnosis, prolonged grief disorder (PGD), has been added to the DSM-5 so adjustment disorder should only be used during the first year or if the person does not meet the criteria for PGD. Changes from DSM-IV to DSM-5 have made the diagnosis of adjustment disorder more useful because, in the previous DSM, it was merely a residual category for distress with symptoms that did not meet criteria for another diagnosis. In the previous criteria, there was no need to identify a precipitating event as there now is. Adjustment disorder also had to resolve much quicker under the DSM-IV whereas with the newest DSM-5-Text Revision (DSM-5-TR), it could be chronic.

ICD-11 Criteria

In the ICD-11, adjustment disorder is distinguished from normal coping responses by intense distress (Maercker & Lorenz, 2018) and reflects a failure to adapt to a normal life stressor. There are also more symptoms included in adjustment disorder: preoccupation with the stressor or its consequences; depressive or anxiety symptoms; as well as increases in maladaptive coping like drinking, smoking, or other substance abuse such that symptoms interfere with everyday functioning like sleep or work. The symptoms usually begin within a month of the onset of the stressor and resolve within six months after the stressor and its consequences have emerged.

Prolonged Grief Disorder

Jim received a telephone call one Thursday evening. He assumed that it was his wife calling to say that she was running late from her job. Jim was eager to talk to his wife because they had fought right before she left for work. He was startled by a male voice who said "Mr. Sojack, could you please come to Mercy Hospital? Your wife is here." He refused to say anything more in response to Jim's questions. When Jim arrived at the emergency room, he was met by two police officers who informed him that his wife had been killed during a robbery.

Eighteen months later, Jim sought out therapy at the urging of his grown children. He had lost 40 pounds, was having problems sleeping, and was barely functioning at work. He had moved out of their bedroom and had left all of his wife's clothing and possessions just as they had been on the night of her death. In one corner of the living room, there was a sort of shrine with a large photograph of his wife, candles, flowers, and a favorite object, a crystal polar bear. Jim informed the therapist that he couldn't really believe she was gone and that he had great guilt over the fight they had the last time he had seen her. He was convinced that she died thinking that he didn't love her. Every time the telephone rang, Jim startled, his heart raced, and he had images of his wife as she had appeared when he identified her body. He felt that his life had lost all meaning.

He was also distressed and angry because the prosecuting attorney was unsure whether the case would ever make it to trial. The evidence was not particularly strong against the two young men who had been arrested, and one of them had withdrawn his confession, which he now said was made under duress. Jim was obsessed with finding out every detail of the crime and often imagined how his wife's last moments must have been for her. After a careful assessment, the therapist diagnosed Jim with prolonged grief disorder and began therapy with him.

DSM-5 Criteria

As everyone knows, the death of a loved one is a great stressor that most people must deal with at some time in their lives. The pandemic that began in 2020 had many journalists discussing grief, especially under the circumstances in which family could not visit the sick person in the hospital or say goodbye, or the helplessness of medical workers who were overwhelmed with deaths and lack of supplies. Grief, the process of mourning the loss of a loved one, is a natural process and is not considered a psychological disorder. The process of grieving and the expected course of bereavement vary from culture to culture. In modern Western culture, people are expected to recover from the death of a loved one far quicker than in the past. Two centuries ago, people were expected to wear particular clothing indicative of mourning for at least a year, a tangible reminder that would serve to elicit the support of others. Queen Victoria was not considered pathological even though she opted for widow's garb for the remainder of her life. However, under the DSM-IV guidelines, a mental health professional could consider a diagnosis of major depression if the symptoms persisted for more than two months, especially if the survivor had strong feelings of guilt, preoccupation with worthlessness, suicidal thoughts, or other symptoms of severe depression.

Diagnosing grief response as pathology has been controversial enough that the *New York Times* took up the gauntlet a number of times between 2010 and 2015 to question whether grief should be considered a disorder. Some of this was because of a change in the definition of depression, which deleted the exclusion of grief from the diagnosis, and there was a concern about medicalizing normal grief. This would result in more older adults being diagnosed with depression. Furthermore, in the meetings of the DSM-5 traumatic stress group, there was no research on the length of time when normal grief becomes abnormal or even what the name of the diagnosis would be. Some called it complicated grief, traumatic grief, or PGD (Simon et al., 2020). The DSM-5 did not include it as a regular disorder but put it in a section called "Conditions for Further Study" to encourage more research. In order to avoid taking sides in what appeared to be an intransigent debate (e.g., Maciejewski et al., 2016; Reynolds et al., 2017), they called it persistent complex bereavement disorder (PCBD). They also set a minimum of 12 months of symptoms, whereas Prigerson et al. (2009) suggested a 6-month starting point. In the 2022 DSM-5-TR, a new disorder of PGD was introduced. It is somewhat different than complicated grief disorder or the PGD that has been suggested previously, does not include anger or survivor's guilt as symptoms, and is different from the ICD-11 PGD.

Box 1.4   Diagnostic Criteria for Prolonged Grief Disorder in DSM-5-TR (F43.8)

Reprinted with permission from Diagnostic and Statistical Manual of Mental Disorders, Fifth Edition, Text Revision (Copyright © 2022). American Psychiatric Association. All Rights Reserved.

A. The death of a person close to the bereaved at least 12 months previously.

B. Since the death, there has been a grief response characterized by one or both of the following, to a clinically significant degree, nearly every day or more often for at least the last month:

    1. Intense yearning/longing for the deceased person.

    2. Preoccupation with thoughts or memories of the deceased person.

C. As a result of the death, at least three of the following eight symptoms have been experienced to a clinically significant degree since the death, including nearly every day or more often for at least the last month:

    1. Identity disruption (e.g., feeling as though part of oneself has died).

    2. Marked sense of disbelief about the death.

    3. Avoidance of reminders that the person is dead.

    4. Intense emotional pain (e.g., anger, bitterness, sorrow) related to the death.

    5. Difficulty with reintegration into life after the death (e.g., problems engaging with friends, pursuing interests, planning for the future).

    6. Emotional numbness.

    7. Feeling that life is meaningless as a result of the death.

    8. Intense loneliness (i.e., feeling alone or detached from others) as a result of the death.

D. The disruption causes clinically significant distress or impairment in social, occupational, or other important areas of functioning.

E. The duration of the bereavement reaction clearly exceeds expected social, cultural, or religious norms for the individual's culture and context.

F. The symptoms are not better explained by major depressive disorder, PTSD, or another mental disorder, or attributable to the physiological effects of a substance (e.g., medication, alcohol) or another medical condition.

So, unlike PTSD in which the person is avoidant of the memories of the traumatic event, the person with PGD is preoccupied by the loss of the loved one for an extended period and has a strong sense of yearning for that person. They have difficulty moving on with their life and have significant disruption in functioning and relating to others as reflected by three of eight symptoms.

ICD-11 Criteria

The ICD-11 criteria also include persistent and pervasive longing and preoccupation with the deceased but are combined with any of ten additional grief reactions (not the three of eight as in the DSM-5-TR). The other symptoms that were added to the ICD-11 include guilt, anger, and blame. The ICD-11 PGD can be diagnosed six months after the loss. However, the ICD-11 advises against diagnosis within the context of some cultural norms for duration of grief response. Some groups expect the grief process to be short, while others prescribe a year of mourning, and still others postpone grief until after the first anniversary of the death. Family and members of the community should be consulted before assuming the grief to be abnormal and in need of diagnosis or treatment.

Although the criteria are different, the name "prolonged grief disorder" was adopted in both the DSM-5-TR and the ICD-11. Although similar to the ICD-11, in response to public comment about pathologizing normal grief as a disorder too soon, the DSM-5-TR version of PGD specifies that it can only be diagnosed after a year has elapsed. In the DSM-5-TR, there can be a delayed response beyond one year, and beyond the core symptoms of intense yearning/longing or preoccupation, the person needs three of eight other symptoms, not any one symptom like the ICD-11.

Summary

Although everyone experiences stress during life, traumatic stress is caused by life-threatening or self-threatening events that are accompanied by a number of specific symptoms. A range of disorders may result from traumatic stressors including adjustment disorder, ASD, PTSD, and PGD. Associated symptoms and disorders may include depression, anxiety disorders, substance abuse, and others. Aside from psychological disorders, traumatic stress may affect some or many areas of a person's functioning, as well as physical health. Future research may tell whether the more inclusive symptoms of the DSM-5 PTSD or the two narrow diagnoses of PTSD and CPTSD from the ICD-11 are going to be more beneficial in identifying those who need help. Because the two diagnoses for PGD are new and still somewhat controversial (Cacciatore & Francis, 2022), it remains to be seen if these disorders are changed over time and what treatments are most beneficial.

References

American Psychiatric Association (1987). *Diagnostic and statistical manual of mental disorders* (3rd ed. Revised; DSM-III-R). Washington D.C.: American Psychiatric Association.

American Psychiatric Association (2013). *Diagnostic and statistical manual of mental disorders* (5th ed.; DSM-5). Washington, D.C.: American Psychiatric Association.

American Psychiatric Association (2022). *Diagnostic and statistical manual of mental disorders* (5th ed-text revision; DSM-5-TR). Washington D.C.: American Psychiatric Association.

Blanchard, E. B., Hickling, E. J., Buckley, T. C., Taylor, A. E., Vollmer, A., & Loos, W. R. (1996). Psychophysiology of posttraumatic stress disorder related to motor vehicle accidents: Replication and extension. *Journal of Consulting and Clinical Psychology, 64,* 742–751.

Brewin, C. R., Cloitre, M., Hyland, P., Shevlin, M., Maercker, A., Bryant, R. A., Humayun, A., Jones, L. M., Kageee, A., Rousseau, C., Somasundaram, D., Suzuki, Y., Wessely, S., van Ommeren, M., & Reed, G. M. (2017). A review of current evidence regarding the ICD-11 proposals for diagnosing PTSD and complex PTSD. *Clinical Psychology Review, 58,* 1–15.

Bryant, R. A., Creamer, M., O'Donnell, M., Silove, D., & McFarland, A. C. (2008). A multisite study of the capacity of acute stress disorder diagnosis to predict posttraumatic stress disorder. *Journal of Clinical Psychiatry, 69,* 923–929.

Bryant, R. A., Friedman, M. J., Spiegel, D., Ursano, R., & Strain, J. (2011). A review of acute stress disorder in DSM-5. *Depression and Anxiety, 28,* 802–817.

Cacciatore, J., & Frances, A. (2022) DSM-5-TR turns normal grief into a mental disorder. *Lancet Psychiatry, 9,* e32.

Friedman, M. J., Resick, P. A., Bryant, R. A., & Brewin, C. R. (2011). Considering PTSD for DSM-5. *Depression and Anxiety,* 750–769.

Green, B., Lindy, J., Grace, M., & Leonard, B. (1992). Chronic Posttraumatic Stress Disorder and diagnostic comorbidity in a disaster sample. *Journal of Nervous and Mental Disease, 180,* 760–766.

Griffin, M. G., Resick, P. A., & Mechanic, M. B. (1997, August). Objective assessment of peritraumatic dissociation: Psychophysiological indicators. *American Journal of Psychiatry, 154,* 1081–1088.

Lanius, R. A., Brand, B. Vermetten, E., Frewen, P. A., & Spiegel, D. (2012). The dissociative subtype of posttraumatic stress disorder: Rationale, clinical and neurobiological evidence, and implications. *Depression and Anxiety, 29,* 701–701.

Lanius, R. A., Vermetten, E., Loewensteiin, R. J., Brand, B., Schmahl, C., Bremner, J. D., & Spiegel, D. (2010). Emotion modulation in PTSD: Clinical and neurobiological evidence for a dissociative subtype. *American Journal of Psychiatry, 167,* 640–647.

Lanius, R. A., Williamson, P. C., Boksman, K., Densmore, M., Gupta, M., Neufeld, R. W. J., Gati, J. S., & Menon, R. S. (2002). Brain activation during script-driven imagery induced dissociative responses in PTSD: A functional magnetic resonance imaging investigation. *Biological Psychiatry, 52,* 305–311.

Maciejewski, P. K., Maercker, A., Boelen, P. A., & Prigerson, H. G. (2016). "Prolonged grief disorder" and "persistent complex bereavement disorder", but not "complicated grief", are one and the same diagnostic entity: An analysis of data from the Yale Bereavement Study. *World Psychiatry, 15,* 266–275.

Maercker, A., & Lorenz, L. (2018). Adjustment disorder diagnosis: Improving clinical utility. *The World Journal of Biological Psychiatry, 19,* 53–513.

Mayou, R., Bryant, B., & Duthie, R. (1993). Psychiatric consequences of road traffic accidents. *British Medical Journal, 307*, 647–651.

McFarlane, A. C. (1988). The longitudinal course of posttraumatic morbidity: The range of outcomes and their predictors. *The Journal of Nervous and Mental Disease, 176*, 30–39.

Monson, C. M., Shnaider, P., Wagner, A. C., Liebman, R. E., Pukey-Martin, N. D., Landy, M. S. H., Wanklyn, S. G., Suvak, M., Hart, T. L., & Koerner, N. (2021). Longitudinal associations between interpersonal relationship functioning and posttraumatic stress disorder (PTSD) in recently traumatized individuals: Differential findings by assessment method. *Psychological Medicine, 53*, 2205–2215.

Norris, F., & Kaniasty, K. (1994). Psychological distress following criminal victimization: Cross-sectional, longitudinal, and prospective analyses. *Journal of Consulting and Clinical Psychology, 10*, 239–261.

Prigerson, H. G., Horowitz, M. J., Jacobs, S. C., Parkes, C. M., Aslan, M., Goodkin, K., Raphael, B., Marwit, S. J., Wortman, C., Neimeyer, R. A., Bonanno, G., Block, S. D., Kissane, D., Boelen, P., Maercker, A., Litz, B. T., Johnson, J. G., First, M. B., & Maciejewski, P. K. (2009). Prolonged grief disorder: Psychometric validation of criteria proposed for DSM-V and ICD-11. *PLoS Medicine, 6*, e1000121.

Resick, P. A., Suvak, M. K., Johnides, B. D., Mitchell, K. S., & Iverson, K. M. (2012). The impact of dissociation on PTSD treatment with Cognitive Processing Therapy. *Depression and Anxiety, 29*, 718–730.

Reynolds, C. F., Cozza, S. J., & Shear, M. K. (2017). Clinically relevant diagnostic criteria for a persistent impairing grief disorder: Putting patients first. *JAMA Psychiatry, 74*(5), 433–434.

Rothbaum, B. O., Foa, E. B., Riggs, D. S., Murdock, T., & Walsh, W. (1992). A prospective examination of post-traumatic stress disorder in rape victims. *Journal of Traumatic Stress, 5*, 455–475.

Simon, N. M., Shear, M. K., Reynolds, C. F., Cozza, S. J., Mauro, C., Zisook, S., Skritskaya, N., Robinaugh, D. J., Malgarroli, M., Spandorfer, J., & Lebowitz, B. (2020). Commentary on evidence in support of a grief-related condition as a DSM diagnosis. *Depression and Anxiety, 37*, 9–16.

Spiegel, D., Koopman, C., Cardeña, E., & Classen, C. (1996). Dissociative symptoms in the diagnosis of acute stress disorder. In W. J. Ray (Ed.), *Handbook of dissociation* (pp. 367–380). New York: Plenum Press.

Wolf, E. J., Miller, M. W., Reardon, A. F., Ryabchenko, K. A., Castillo, D., & Freund, R. (2012). A latent class analysis of dissociation and posttraumatic stress disorder: Evidence for a dissociative subtype. *Archives of General Psychiatry, 69*, 698–703.

Wolf, E. J., Mitchell, K. S., Sadeh, N., Hein, C., Fuhrman, I., Pietrzak, R. H., & Miller, M.W. (2017). The dissociative subtype of PTSD Scale: Initial evaluation in a national sample of trauma-exposed veterans. *Assessment, 24*, 503–516.

World Health Organization (2019). *International statistical classification of diseases and related health problems* (11th ed.). https://icd.who.int/

2

Prevalence of Traumatic Events and Trauma- and Stressor-Related Disorders

A century or two ago, life expectancies were lower than they are now, infant and maternal mortality were higher, antibiotics had not been discovered, bad weather could not be predicted with any accuracy, and workplace safety practices had not been established. People did not openly discuss family violence, sexual assault, or incest. People did not work in offices behind computers, but much more commonly worked in factories, mines, and farms. Today, people in industrialized countries do not necessarily expect that sudden catastrophic events can or will happen to them. The purpose of this chapter will be to describe the prevalence of traumatic events and the frequency with which people develop psychological disorders such as posttraumatic stress disorder (PTSD) in response to them.

Within the topic of traumatic stress, prevalence can be examined on several different levels. First, it is possible to examine how frequently stressful/traumatic events occur to people within a given period of time or across their lifetime. Aside from determining the frequency of traumatic stressors in people's lives, it is also possible to determine the frequency of various psychological outcomes—the prevalence of psychological problems in the aftermath of trauma. These outcomes could be examined singly or in combination. The co-occurrence of more than one diagnosable disorder is referred to as "comorbidity". This chapter will provide an overview of the prevalence of traumatic stressors in people's lives and will then summarize the prevalence of diagnosable disorders following traumatic events. Finally, the comorbidity of disorders will be discussed.

DOI: 10.4324/9780429317934-2

Prevalence of Trauma

Although most people regularly experience stress and daily hassles, traumatic events, by their very nature, are rarer. That is to say, traumatic events are not common daily experiences in most people's lives. Some people never experience trauma in their lifetimes. However, the majority of people will experience at least one traumatic event, and a large number will experience more than one of these major events, in their lifetime.

Many traumas are crimes and therefore trackable by crime surveys and databases. In the United States, two of the major criminal victimization surveys, which are conducted annually, are the National Crime Victimization Survey and the Uniform Crime Reports. The National Crime Victimization Survey is a survey of 150,000 households and considers a range of crimes that may or may not have been reported to the police. The Uniform Crime Reports consider those crimes that were reported to police. According to the National Crime Victimization Survey, in 2021, only 46% of violent victimizations were reported to the police. Both of these surveys break down crime rates by a variety of demographic variables (Thompson & Tapp, 2022).

Victimization incidence is calculated as the number of victimizations divided by the number of persons/households in a specific category of interest. According to the US National Crime Victimization Survey, in 2021, for every 1,000 people aged 12 and older, there were 1.2 rapes, 2.7 aggravated assaults, and 1.7 robberies. It should be noted that criminal victimization is only one type of traumatic stressor that could affect people. Combat trauma, accidents, natural disasters, and political terrorism/war are all significant traumas that may contribute to psychological problems.

In contrast to incidence, prevalence is the number of persons or households who have been victimized one or more times in a given time period divided by the population of interest. It is, therefore, the percentage of people who have experienced trauma in the population. The period of time could be a single year, or it could be across the course of a lifetime. When the prevalence of disorders is examined, it can also be presented as the percentage of people who experience the disorder at some point in their lives or the percentage of people who are currently experiencing the disorder. The prevalence of trauma has been estimated based on national surveys with the general population and with specific populations, such as veterans. Prevalence estimates suggest that exposure to one or more traumatic events in one's lifetime is extremely common.

The National Comorbidity Study (Kessler et al., 1995) was the first comprehensive study of trauma and PTSD (and many other psychological disorders) in the general population. Kessler et al. surveyed a representative national sample of 5,877 persons (2,812 men and 3,065 women) in the United States and assessed

12 categories of traumatic events. They found that a majority of people had experienced at least one major traumatic event. In that sample, more than 60% of men and 51% of women reported exposure to at least one trauma, and most had experienced multiple traumas. This study found that of those who had experienced trauma, only a little over a quarter of the sample reported experiencing only one major trauma; 15% of the men and 14% of the women reported experiencing two; 10% of the men and 5% of the women had experienced three; and another 10% of men and 6% of women reported four major traumas. So, overall, 35% of the men and 25% of the women reported more than one traumatic event in their lives thus far. While the majority of people in that study reported experiencing at least one traumatic event, there was a great deal of variability in what types of events were experienced. The most common events were witnessing someone seriously injured or killed, disasters, and accidents. Experience with these events was reported by 19–36% of the men and 14–15% of the women. Less commonly reported were rapes, physical assaults, and child abuse. However, there have been more recent studies and studies that have focused on these latter topics in particular that have shown higher rates, perhaps because these more sensitive topics need special attention during survey questioning. Although there has been improvement in how we ask people about trauma exposure, it is quite possible that people don't apply the words "rape", "assault", or "abuse" to themselves, especially when these events are perpetrated by acquaintances or family. There are also data suggesting that studies using longer lists of traumas report higher lifetime exposure rates (Kessler et al., 2022). Thus, a number of methodological factors may impact endorsement of traumatic events and therefore recorded prevalence rates.

Kilpatrick et al. (2013) conducted the National Stressful Events Survey, indicated a significantly higher rate of trauma exposure. In this study, 90% of US respondents reported exposure to at least one Diagnostic and Statistical Manual of Mental Disorders, Fifth Edition (DSM-5) traumatic event. The modal number of events experienced was three. The most commonly reported traumas were assaults, deaths of others, disasters, and accidents (see Table 2.1).

Similarly, in a national probability sample of the general population of Norwegian adults, lifetime exposure was 85% in men and 86% in women (Heir et al., 2019). The average number of categories of traumatic events experienced was four, and most respondents (27%) experienced four to six different event categories. The most common events experienced were transportation accidents (45%) and life-threatening illness or injury (49%). Men were more likely to report experiencing natural disasters, fire or explosions, transportation accidents, and other serious accidents, whereas women were more likely to report experiencing sexual assault, other unwanted or uncomfortable sexual experiences, life-threatening illness or injury, human suffering, sudden violent deaths, and "other" stressful events.

Table 2.1 National Stressful Events Survey: Weighted prevalence of DSM-5 Criterion A traumatic events, in order of associated lifetime prevalence of PTSD (Kilpatrick et al. 2013)

Traumatic Event	Prevalence of Event (%)	Prevalence of PTSD Secondary to Event (%)
Sexual/physical assault	53.1	7.3
Death due to violence/accident/disaster	51.8	4.3
Combat/war-zone exposure	7.8	3.8
Family/close friend threat/injury	32.4	2.5
Witnessing sexual/physical assault	33.2	1.8
Witnessing dead bodies	22.6	1.4
Hazardous chemical exposure	16.7	1.0
Accident/fire	48.3	0.9
Disaster	50.5	0.4
Work/secondary exposure	11.5	0.2

Trauma Exposure Across Countries

The World Health Organization's World Mental Health Surveys included a series of population studies that estimated the prevalence of traumatic events across 24 countries on 6 continents including 14 high-income countries, 7 upper-middle-income countries, and 6 low/lower-middle-income countries. Results indicated that across countries, 70.4% of respondents experienced at least one traumatic event, although prevalence varied widely across countries from 28.6% to 84.6% (Benjet et al., 2016). Variation in the trauma exposure rates and rates of specific traumatic events by country might reflect different historical, cultural, or political factors (Atwoli et al., 2015).

With respect to the number of traumatic events experienced, multiple trauma exposures were the norm, with 18.2% experiencing one event, 12.7% experiencing two, 9.1% experiencing three, and 30.5% experiencing four or more. The most common category of events was accidents/injuries (36.3%), and the most common single event type was unexpected death of a loved one (31.4%), followed by witnessing death, a dead body, or someone seriously injured (23.7%); being mugged (14.5%); and life-threatening automobile accidents (14.0%).

A number of sociodemographic factors predicted trauma exposure across these surveys. It was observed that women were more than twice as likely to experience intimate partner/sexual violence and slightly more likely to experience unexpected death of a loved one. Men, on the other hand, were more likely to be exposed to most other traumas. Younger age was generally associated with greater trauma exposure. Married respondents were less likely to experience most trauma categories except accidents/injuries. Correlates of trauma exposure also varied by country, potentially reflecting different sociopolitical contexts (Atwoli et al., 2015).

Trauma Exposure Among Veterans

Military veterans have particularly high rates of trauma exposure and PTSD and are therefore an important population to consider with respect to prevalence. The National Health and Resilience in Veterans Study was a web-based survey of a nationally representative population-based sample of US veterans. In this sample, 87% of veterans reported exposure to at least one traumatic event, and the mean number of events was three (Wisco et al., 2014). Most common were sudden death of a close family member or friend (61%), witnessing death or injury (38%), combat (34%), natural disasters (34%), and life-threatening illness or injury (30%).

Clearly, a large majority of the population has experienced at least one traumatic event. However, not all people suffer from psychological disorders as a result of these traumas.

Prevalence of Trauma- and Stressor-Related Disorders

There are many ways in which people might be affected by their traumatic experiences. They may display a pattern of resilience, with little to no change in functioning. They may initially experience distress but recover from the experience fully with no measurable psychological, biological, or behavioral consequences. Or they may develop a diagnosable psychological disorder that may be experienced briefly or over a long period of time.

Some studies have examined different response trajectories. Pietrzak et al. (2014) conducted a longitudinal examination of responders to the 9/11 World Trade Center attack over eight years including 4,035 professional police responders and 6,800 nontraditional responders such as construction workers, maintenance, and other heterogeneous workers. Among the police responders, there were four PTSD symptom trajectories: resistant/resilient (78%), chronic (5%), recovering (8%), or delayed onset (8.5%). The nontraditional responders had six trajectories: resistant/resilient (58%), recovering (12%), severe chronic (9.5%), subsyndromal increasing (7%), delayed onset (7%), and moderate chronic (6%). The "resilient" groups had low PTSD scores across three assessment points; severe or moderate "chronic" groups had elevated scores that didn't improve over time. Two groups, "subsyndomal increasing" and "delayed onset", showed worsening scores, but the first group did not increase as much as the delayed onset. The biggest difference was that the police responders were much less likely to have PTSD at any point in time than the more heterogeneous nontraditional group of responders. Among both groups, there were predictors of response trajectory. Hispanic ethnicity, psychiatric history, severity of exposure, and event-related medical conditions were most strongly associated with symptomatic trajectories, while more education and family and work support appeared protective.

Lowe et al. (2021) studied trajectories of PTSD symptoms over three or more time points within the first year post-trauma among 3,083 adults admitted to emergency departments for injuries in a multicountry consortium. They found five symptom trajectories: low (64.5%), remitting (16.9%), moderate (6.7%), high (6.5%), and delayed (5.5%). Female gender, non-White race, assaultive injuries, and prior interpersonal traumas were associated with initial PTSD reaction. Those reporting assaultive injuries were at increased risk of both immediate and long-term symptoms. Both of these studies demonstrate that resilience and low symptom burden are common responses following trauma, whereas a subset of individuals experience trauma-related symptoms.

When people are affected, they can experience reactions that impact their interpersonal functioning, such as marital relationships, sexual functioning, family functioning, or ability to form or maintain friendships. Trauma may affect people's relationship with themselves, that is, with regard to self-esteem, confidence, trust in their own judgment, or other beliefs about themselves. Reactions to trauma may compromise the immune system resulting in physical illnesses. Many of these problems were listed in Chapter 1.

To begin the discussion of the prevalence of trauma-related problems, we will primarily discuss PTSD because it is the disorder that appears to develop most frequently and has been studied the most. We will also touch upon acute stress disorder, adjustment disorder, and prolonged grief disorder. However, it is important to note that not all people exposed to trauma experience a psychological disorder, and there are other disorders outside of the trauma- and stressor-related disorders category, such as depression, that people may suffer from following traumatic event exposure.

Posttraumatic Stress Disorder

There are two ways in which the prevalence of PTSD can be examined. One way is to estimate the prevalence across the population as a whole. However, because PTSD requires a trauma to occur before even considering diagnosis, another way is to examine the conditional probability of PTSD, which is the prevalence of PTSD among only those individuals who have experienced a traumatic event.

The National Comorbidity Study (Kessler et al., 1995) was the first systematic epidemiological report of PTSD prevalence. Kessler et al. surveyed 2,812 men and 3,065 women. They found the population prevalence of PTSD to be 7.8% overall, with 10.4% of women and 5% of men having experienced PTSD during their lifetime. The PTSD rate among those exposed to trauma was higher: 20% for women and 8% for men. This study did not examine current PTSD but lifetime PTSD. In discussing the sex difference in PTSD, Kessler et al. pointed out that, whereas men were more likely than women to experience at least one trauma overall, women were more likely than men to experience a trauma associated with a high probability of PTSD (e.g., sexual assault). In the National Comorbidity Study replication study (Kessler et al., 2005), lifetime prevalence of PTSD was estimated similarly at 6.8%. Subsequent studies have also reported similar prevalence rates, although surveys in populations or regions particularly affected by violence have been higher (e.g., Alpak et al., 2015; de Jong et al., 2001).

More recently, using the DSM-5 PTSD criteria, the 2012–2013 National Epidemiologic Survey on Alcohol and Related Conditions-III showed among a nationally representative sample of US civilians a past-year prevalence of PTSD of 4.7% and a lifetime prevalence of 6.1% (Goldstein et al., 2016). In another recent national sample of a demographically and geographically representative panel of US adults, the National Stressful Events Survey showed a 4.7% past-year prevalence, but a slightly higher 8.3% lifetime prevalence of PTSD.

Lifetime prevalence of PTSD also varies by country. For example, the World Mental Health surveys examined prevalence to a randomly selected traumatic event rather than the worst event, which is a methodological strategy to avoid overestimation of PTSD prevalence, to generate more accurate population-level statistics, and to improve cross-country comparisons (Atwoli et al., 2015). As with trauma exposure, there was notable variability between countries. For example, respondents in Northerrn Ireland had higher rates of PTSD (8.8%) compared to Japan (1.8%; Atwoli et al., 2015)

PTSD Prevalence as a Function of Trauma Type

It is clear from the existing research that all traumatic events are not equal, and PTSD rates vary greatly by trauma type. Referring back to Table 2.1, it can be seen that the most common traumatic events are not necessarily the most likely to lead to PTSD. For example, although disasters and accidents are among the most commonly experienced traumas, they are relatively unlikely to lead to PTSD. Of course, such events vary greatly in severity, which may contribute to variability in PTSD symptomatology. Events like sexual and physical assault are more likely to produce PTSD. Rape is the single event most likely to cause PTSD in both men and women. It appears that events that are violent and intended are much more likely to cause PTSD than events that are traumatic but natural, or at least impersonal (accidents). In the National Epidemiologic Survey on Alcohol and Related Conditions-III survey, prevalence of PTSD was highest for interpersonal violence traumas (i.e., 7% for sexual or physical assault) and combat (4%). Also, the more traumas experienced, the more likely someone was to have PTSD. Likewise, in the aforementioned Norwegian study, the most common events causing PTSD were sexual assaults, physical assaults, life-threatening illness or injury, and sudden violent deaths; most often events causing PTSD were experienced personally (64.3%). Again, risk of PTSD increased proportionally with number of event categories reported.

Whether prevalence estimates are based on the worst traumatic event or random traumatic events affects estimates. As noted earlier, a preferred methodological approach that is thought to produce less biased prevalence rates is to base estimates of PTSD on a randomly selected trauma (Breslau et al., 2004). The World Mental Health surveys assessed PTSD prevalence using this approach. In this case, the weighted PTSD prevalence was 4%; however, again, as in other studies, prevalence varied by trauma type. Rape had the highest conditional probability at 19%, followed by physical abuse by a romantic partner (12%) and kidnapping (11%; Liu et al., 2017).

Although the results of these studies are not identical, they are remarkably similar. Overall, it can be estimated that 6–8% of the US population have experienced diagnosable PTSD at some time in their lives. Among other countries, rates vary, but many fall in this same range. These percentages may appear small, but they translate to millions of people on a national or international scale.

Among veterans exposed to combat, the conditional probability of PTSD has been estimated at 12.1% (Wisco et al., 2014). Risk also varied as a function of the degree of combat exposure: Moderate-to-heavy and heavy combat exposure was associated with greater PTSD risk (25–35%). Although sexual abuse was infrequently endorsed in the veteran sample, these traumas were associated with some of the highest conditional probabilities of PTSD (26–37%), consistent with the civilian literature.

Prospective Studies of PTSD Following Trauma Exposure

Most of the studies described previously are retrospective studies. A retrospective study assesses the prevalence of trauma and/or disorders across a particular population regarding events that happened at some time in the past. Although some studies have a fairly short time frame such as events occurring in the past year, many prevalence studies ask participants to report on events or symptoms across their whole lifetime. The advantage of retrospective population studies is that the sample may be very representative of the population of interest. The disadvantage is that trauma reactions are being questioned and compiled for events that may have occurred perhaps decades apart and could be affected by memory and subsequent events.

A prospective study assesses participants' reactions from the time of a traumatic event forward for some period of time. The advantage of this type of study is that everyone is assessed at uniform times post-trauma so the reactions are not affected by time, nor are they affected as much by memory and recall as retrospective studies. However, because the participants must have told someone about the incident in order to be identified and invited to participate in the research, these studies cannot be assumed to represent the population as a whole. For example, people who do not report their victimization to someone might have different types or severity of reactions from those who report and discuss their trauma with others.

One prospective study by Rothbaum et al. (1992) assessed PTSD weekly in 95 rape victims after they reported their crimes to the police/hospital. They found that at the first assessment (average time was 13 days post-crime), 94% of the women met the symptom criteria for PTSD; 12 weeks later, 47% had full PTSD. In a similar study with male and female nonsexual assault victims who were victimized by nonfamily members (robbery, simple assault, aggravated assault), the researchers found a similar but less severe pattern of recovery (Riggs et al., 1995). At the first assessment, within a month of the crime, 71% of the women and 50% of the men met the symptom criteria for PTSD. At the final assessment, 12 weeks later, 21% of the 38 women and none of the 22 men who completed the study had PTSD. Riggs et al. pointed out that although many of the participants did not have full PTSD at the final assessment, many of them still had component symptoms. More than 50% of the non-PTSD participants met the reexperiencing and arousal criteria, although few reported sufficient avoidance/numbing symptoms to meet the avoidance criteria or the overall diagnostic criteria. They also found that those who dropped out of the study (i.e., did not complete all of the assessments) reported more severe assaults than those who completed the study. The authors concluded that their rates of PTSD might be an underestimate of the true level of reactions following assault.

These studies are informative because they highlight how after a traumatic event, not everyone goes on to meet criteria for PTSD—even if they initially experience PTSD symptoms. It is important to remember that it's more common for people to experience resilience or natural recovery from traumatic events than to develop PTSD. These data also highlight that similar patterns of recovery occur for different trauma types; however, rates of symptoms vary by trauma, consistent with cross-sectional research indicating that some trauma types such as sexual assault are more likely to produce PTSD symptoms.

Other Trauma-Related Disorders

Of the trauma- and stressor-related disorders, the prevalence of PTSD has been estimated in large, general population studies, whereas population-based studies of other trauma-related disorders have been scant or nonexistent. However, smaller studies and studies focused on specific groups of trauma-affected individuals have been used to estimate the prevalence of these other disorders. Because these studies are not necessarily representative of the population as a whole, the estimates should be interpreted more cautiously.

Acute Stress Disorder

Rates of acute stress disorder have varied widely in the literature. For example, rates have ranged from 9% among motor vehicle accident victims (Hamanaka et al., 2006) to 69% among sexual assault victims (Armour et al., 2013). Estimates of acute stress disorder even vary widely within trauma types, such as estimates of acute stress disorder following natural disasters (5–62%; Lavenda et al., 2017; Mills et al., 2007). Most currently available estimates of acute stress disorder prevalence are based on earlier versions of the DSM. Bryant et al. (2015, see Chapter 1) found that rates may be higher with DSM-5, consistent with easier-to-meet inclusion criteria for the diagnosis in the most recent classification system. As with PTSD, closer proximity to the traumatic event is associated with increased risk of acute stress disorder (Blanchard et al., 2004).

Adjustment Disorder

Prevalence of adjustment disorder has been examined in a few population-based studies, and rates have been very low (<1–2%). This was the case in one study across five European countries and two studies in Germany (Carta et al., 2009; Glaesmer et al., 2015; Maercker et al., 2012). However, rates of adjustment disorder have been higher when examined in specific populations such as those with recent job loss or recently bereaved (18–27%; Killikelly et al., 2019; Perkonigg et al., 2018). The wide range of estimates for acute stress disorder and adjustment disorder highlights potential methodological differences that may influence estimates. As with PTSD, adjustment disorder is more common among women than among men (Gradus et al., 2022).

Prolonged Grief Disorder

Prevalence estimates for prolonged grief disorder are lacking due to the novelty of this specific diagnosis as currently conceptualized in the DSM-5-TR and International Classification of Diseases, 11th Edition (ICD-11). A meta-analysis based on earlier prolonged grief definitions produced a pooled conditional prevalence of 9.8% (Lundorff et al., 2017). In another meta-analysis of prolonged grief disorder following deaths by nonnatural causes such as homicides and accidents, a pooled prevalence of 49% was observed (Djelantik et al., 2020). Thus, there is clearly great variability in estimates, based on population, loss type, and likely other methodological factors such as the questions asked to determine the presence of prolonged grief. In a representative sample in Germany, Rosner et al. (2021) reported the prevalence of the current diagnostic criteria for prolonged grief disorder was 1–2% in the total sample and 3–4% among bereaved individuals, with lower prevalence for DSM-5 versus ICD-11.

Comorbidity of Trauma-Related Disorders

Because other trauma- and stressor-related disorders have been studied less, most research has attended to the prevalence of comorbidities with PTSD. Comorbidity is the co-occurrence of more than one diagnosable disorder. It is possible that other disorders develop independently of PTSD. However, it is also possible that other disorders develop as maladaptive coping attempts in response to trauma and PTSD symptoms and then become full-blown problems in and of themselves. For example, if someone has severe PTSD symptoms including nightmares, sleep disruption, flash-backs, hypervigilance, and other physiological arousal symptoms, that person may attempt to reduce their symptomatology by consuming alcohol. If the person con-sumes enough alcohol to become addicted or to cause serious problems in their life, then they would also have an alcohol use disorder diagnosis secondary to the PTSD. If the person had an alcohol use disorder prior to the trauma, then both the alcohol use disorder and PTSD might be primary diagnoses.

An example of an epidemiological study is the aforementioned National Comor-bidity Study in which Kessler et al. (1995) conducted a national survey of 5,877 people. They found that of those with PTSD, 88% of the men and 79% of the women also had comorbid disorders. Table 2.2 lists the most common comorbid disorders for men and women.

More recent estimates are consistent in finding that psychiatric comorbidities are extremely common, with upward of 70% of those with PTSD also having another comorbid diagnosis. Estimates suggest 35–52% of those with PTSD meet criteria for major depressive disorder, 36–59% meet criteria for anxiety disorders, and 25–46% meet criteria for alcohol use disorder (Crum-Cianflone et al., 2016; Pietrzak et al., 2011; Rytwinski et al., 2013; Walter et al., 2018).

In thinking about the meaning of these findings, it is clear that the rates of comor-bid disorders are very high. Relatively few people suffer from only one disorder such as PTSD. Most of those with PTSD also develop one or more other diagnosable disor-ders. Epidemiological studies help to characterize the prevalence of comorbid disorders

Table 2.2 Prevalence of disorders comorbid with PTSD in the National Comorbidity Study (Kessler et al., 1995)

	Men (%)	Women (%)
Major depressive disorder	48	49
Dysthymia	21	23
Mania	12	6
Generalized anxiety disorder	17	15
Panic	7	13
Simple phobia	31	29
Social phobia	28	28
Agoraphobia	16	22
Alcohol	52	28
Drugs	35	27
Conduct disorder	43	15

across the population and over one's lifetime. However, it should be noted again that community surveys are retrospective studies in which some participants are reporting about events and symptoms that may have occurred years or even decades earlier, whereas other participants may have experienced traumatic events more recently. These studies also report across a range of potential traumatic events that could vary a great deal in their likelihood of producing PTSD or other comorbid disorders. Given that epidemiological studies assess disorders across a lifetime, it is possible that the rates of comorbidity are higher than one would find if they examined participants cross-sectionally, that is, at a specific time after a traumatic event happens.

Summary

Although not frequent in daily life, most people experience at least one traumatic event over the course of their lives—most studies indicate that upward of 70% of the population experience at least one traumatic stressor during their lifetime, and most experience multiple traumas. In the general population, 6–8% have suffered from diagnosable PTSD, though there are typically sex differences reported, with women having higher rates than men. There is a great deal of variability in rates of PTSD depending upon the type of trauma and across countries. Interpersonal violence is most likely to lead to PTSD. PTSD occurs very frequently with other disorders, most commonly major depression. Fortunately, as you will read in Chapter 7 on treatment, there are many effective treatments for PTSD and comorbid issues.

References

Alpak, G., Unal, A., Bulbul, F., Sagaltici, E., Bez, Y., Altindag, A., Dalkilic, A., & Savas, H. A. (2015). Post-traumatic stress disorder among Syrian refugees in Turkey: A cross-sectional study. *International Journal of Psychiatry in Clinical Practice, 19*(1), 45–50.

Armour, C., Elklit, A., & Shevlin, M. (2013). The latent structure of acute stress disorder: A posttraumatic stress disorder approach. *Psychological Trauma: Theory, Research, Practice, and Policy, 5*(1), 18–25.

Atwoli, L., Stein, D. J., Koenen, K. C., & McLaughlin, K. A. (2015). Epidemiology of post-traumatic stress disorder: Prevalence, correlates and consequences. *Current Opinion in Psychiatry, 28*(4), 307–322.

Benjet, C., Bromet, E., Karam, E. G., Kessler, R. C., McLaughlin, K. A., Ruscio, A. M.,... & Koenen, K. C. (2016). The epidemiology of traumatic event exposure worldwide: Results from the World Mental Health Survey Consortium. *Psychological Medicine, 46*(2), 327–343.

Blanchard, E. B., Kuhn, E., Rowell, D. L., Hickling, E. J., Wittrock, D., Rogers, R. L.,... & Steckler, D. C. (2004). Studies of the vicarious traumatization of college students by the September 11th attacks: Effects of proximity, exposure and connectedness. *Behaviour Research and Therapy, 42*(2), 191–205.

Breslau, N., Peterson, E. L., Poisson, L. M., Schultz, L. R., & Lucia, V. C. (2004). Estimating post-traumatic stress disorder in the community: Lifetime perspective and the impact of typical traumatic events. *Psychological Medicine, 34*(5), 889–898.

Bryant, R. A., Creamer, M., O'Donnell, M., Silove, D., McFarlane, A. C., & Forbes, D. (2015). A comparison of the capacity of DSM-IV and DSM-5 acute stress disorder definitions to predict posttraumatic stress disorder and related disorders. *The Journal of Clinical Psychiatry, 76*(4), 3467.

Carta, M. G., Balestrieri, M., Murru, A., & Hardoy, M. C. (2009). Adjustment disorder: Epidemiology, diagnosis and treatment. *Clinical Practice and Epidemiology in Mental Health, 5*(1), 1–15.

Crum-Cianflone, N. F., Powell, T. M., LeardMann, C. A., Russell, D. W., & Boyko, E. J. (2016). Mental health and comorbidities in US military members. *Military Medicine, 181*(6), 537–545.

De Jong, J. T., Komproe, I. H., Van Ommeren, M., El Masri, M., Araya, M., Khaled, N., van de Put, W., & Somasundaram, D. (2001). Lifetime events and posttraumatic stress disorder in 4 postconflict settings. *JAMA, 286*(5), 555–562.

Djelantik, A.A.A. M. J., Smid, G., E., Mroz, A., Kleber, R.J., Boelen, P.A. (2020). The prevalence of prolonged grief disorder in bereaved individuals following unnatural losses: Systematic review and meta regression analysis. *Journal of Affective Disorders*, 265, 146–156.

Glaesmer, H., Romppel, M., Brähler, E., Hinz, A., & Maercker, A. (2015). Adjustment disorder as proposed for ICD-11: Dimensionality and symptom differentiation. *Psychiatry Research, 229*(3), 940–948.

Goldstein, R. B., Smith, S. M., Chou, S. P., Saha, T. D., Jung, J., Zhang, H., Pickering, R. P., Ruan, W. J., Huang, B., & Grant, B. F. (2016). The epidemiology of DSM-5 posttraumatic stress disorder in the United States: Results from the National Epidemiologic Survey on Alcohol and Related Conditions-III. *Social Psychiatry and Psychiatric Epidemiology, 51*, 1137–1148.

Gradus, J. L., Rosellini, A. J., Szentkúti, P., Horváth-Puhó, E., Smith, M. L., Galatzer-Levy, I.,... & Sørensen, H. T. (2022). Using Danish national registry data to understand psychopathology following potentially traumatic experiences. *Journal of Traumatic Stress, 35*(2), 619–630.

Hamanaka, S., Asukai, N., Kamijo, Y., Hatta, K., Kishimoto, J., & Miyaoka, H. (2006). Acute stress disorder and posttraumatic stress disorder symptoms among patients severely injured in motor vehicle accidents in Japan. *General Hospital Psychiatry, 28*(3), 234–241.

Heir, T., Bonsaksen, T., Grimholt, T., Ekeberg, Ø., Skogstad, L., Lerdal, A., & Schou-Bredal, I. (2019). Serious life events and post-traumatic stress disorder in the Norwegian population. *BJPsych Open, 5*(5), e82.

Kessler, R. C., Benjet, C., Bromet, E. J., & Rosellini, A. J. (2022). The epidemiology of PTSD among adults. In J. G. Beck & D. M. Sloan (Eds.), *The Oxford handbook of traumatic stress disorders* (2nd ed., pp. 126–154). New York: Oxford University Press.

Kessler, R. C., Berglund, P., Demler, O., Jin, R., Merikangas, K. R., & Walters, E. E. (2005). Lifetime prevalence and age-of-onset distributions of DSM-IV disorders in the National Comorbidity Survey Replication. *Archives of General Psychiatry, 62*(6), 593–602.

Kessler, R. C., Sonnega, A., Bromet, E., Hughes, M., & Nelson, C. B. (1995). Posttraumatic stress disorder in the National Comorbidity Survey. *Archives of General Psychiatry, 52*(12), 1048–1060.

Killikelly, C., Lorenz, L., Bauer, S., Mahat-Shamir, M., Ben-Ezra, M., & Maercker, A. (2019). Prolonged grief disorder: Its co-occurrence with adjustment disorder and post-traumatic stress disorder in a bereaved Israeli general-population sample. *Journal of Affective Disorders, 249*, 307–314.

Kilpatrick, D. G., Resnick, H. S., Milanak, M. E., Miller, M. W., Keyes, K. M., & Friedman, M. J. (2013). National estimates of exposure to traumatic events and PTSD prevalence using DSM-IV and DSM-5 criteria. *Journal of Traumatic Stress, 26*(5), 537–547.

Lavenda, O., Grossman, E. S., Ben-Ezra, M., & Hoffman, Y. (2017). Exploring DSM-5 criterion A in acute stress disorder symptoms following natural disaster. *Psychiatry Research, 256*, 458–460.

Liu, H., Petukhova, M. V., Sampson, N. A., Aguilar-Gaxiola, S., Alonso, J., Andrade, L. H.,… & World Health Organization World Mental Health Survey Collaborators. (2017). Association of DSM-IV posttraumatic stress disorder with traumatic experience type and history in the World Health Organization World Mental Health Surveys. *JAMA Psychiatry, 74*(3), 270–281.

Lowe S. R., Ratanatharathorn, A., Lai, B. S., van der Mei, W., Barbano, A. C., Bryant, R. A., Delahanty, D. L., Matsuoka, Y. J., Olff, M., Schnyder, U., Laska, E., Koenen, K.C., Shalev, A. Y., & Kessler, R. C. (2021). Posttraumatic stress disorder symptom trajectories within the first year following emergency department admissions: Pooled results from the International Consortium to predict PTSD. *Psychological Medicine, 51,* 1129–1139.

Lundorff, M., Holmgren, H., Zachariae, R., Farver-Vestergaard, I., & O'Connor, M. (2017). Prevalence of prolonged grief disorder in adult bereavement: A systematic review and meta-analysis. *Journal of Affective Disorders, 212*, 138–149.

Maercker, A., Forstmeier, S., Pielmaier, L., Spangenberg, L., Brähler, E., & Glaesmer, H. (2012). Adjustment disorders: Prevalence in a representative nationwide survey in Germany. *Social Psychiatry and Psychiatric Epidemiology, 47*, 1745–1752.

Mills, M. A., Edmondson, D., & Park, C. L. (2007). Trauma and stress response among Hurricane Katrina evacuees. *American Journal of Public Health, 97*(Supplement_1), S116–S123.

Perkonigg, A., Lorenz, L., & Maercker, A. (2018). Prevalence and correlates of ICD-11 adjustment disorder: Findings from the Zurich Adjustment Disorder Study. *International Journal of Clinical and Health Psychology, 18*(3), 209–217.

Pietrzak, R. H., Feder, A., Singh, R., Schechter, C. B., Bromet, E. J., Katz, C. L., Reissman, D. B., Ozbay, F., Sharma, V., Crane, M., Harrison, D., Herbert, R., Levin, S. M., Luft B. J., Moline, J. M., Stellman, J. M., Udasin, I. G., Landrigan, P. J., & Southwick, S. M., (2014). Trajectories of PTSD risk and resilience in World Trade Center responders: An 8-year prospective cohort study. *Psychological Medicine, 44*, 205–219.

Pietrzak, R. H., Goldstein, R. B., Southwick, S. M., & Grant, B. F. (2011). Prevalence and Axis I comorbidity of full and partial posttraumatic stress disorder in the United States: Results from Wave 2 of the National Epidemiologic Survey on Alcohol and Related Conditions. *Journal of Anxiety Disorders, 25*(3), 456–465.

Riggs, D. S., Rothbaum, B. O., & Foa, E. B. (1995). A prospective examination of symptoms of posttraumatic stress disorder in victims of nonsexual assault. *Journal of Interpersonal Violence, 10*(2), 201–214.

Rosner, R., Comtesse, H., Vogel, A., & Doering, B. K. (2021). Prevalence of prolonged grief disorder. *Journal of Affective Disorders, 287*, 301–307.

Rothbaum, B. O., Foa, E. B., Riggs, D. S., Murdock, T., & Walsh, W. (1992). A prospective examination of post-traumatic stress disorder in rape victims. *Journal of Traumatic Stress, 5*(3), 455–475.

Rytwinski, N. K., Scur, M. D., Feeny, N. C., & Youngstrom, E. A. (2013). The co-occurrence of major depressive disorder among individuals with posttraumatic stress disorder: A meta-analysis. *Journal of Traumatic Stress, 26*(3), 299–309.

Thompson, A., & Tapp, S. N. (2022). Criminal Victimization, 2021, Bureau of Justice Statistics. Accessed from: https://bjs.ojp.gov/library/publications/criminal-victimization-2021

Walter, K. H., Levine, J. A., Highfill-McRoy, R. M., Navarro, M., & Thomsen, C. J. (2018). Prevalence of posttraumatic stress disorder and psychological comorbidities among US active duty service members, 2006–2013. *Journal of Traumatic Stress, 31*(6), 837–844.

Wisco, B. E., Marx, B. P., Wolf, E. J., Miller, M. W., Southwick, S. M., & Pietrzak, R. H. (2014). Posttraumatic stress disorder in the US veteran population: Results from the National Health and Resilience in Veterans Study. *The Journal of Clinical Psychiatry, 75*(12), 14904.

3

Psychological Theories of Traumatic Stress

Theories are the skeletons upon which we produce an understanding of the phenomenon under consideration. A good theory should explain and account for the findings from research. In fact, if research findings contradict or do not support a theory, then the theory should be modified or discarded. A good theory of trauma response should be able to describe the reactions that have been observed clinically, increase our ability to predict who will develop problems (or not), and point to the elements of effective treatment. A good theory should be testable and lead to a logical series of studies to examine the topic of interest.

Throughout the history of psychology, there have been large periods of time in which trauma was largely ignored and no research was conducted. There have been times of increased awareness, particularly in times of war, during which theories, clinical attention, and research increased dramatically, only to be neglected once the war ceased. However, in the late 1970s and 1980s, attention increased from several different arenas (the Vietnam war, the women's rights movement, attention to child abuse, the victim assistance movement, disaster work), and research interests converged and expanded beyond what had ever existed previously. As a result, research has proliferated into an entire field of study, and theories have been offered to explain the findings. Although there are some older theories, this chapter will mostly cover more recent theories of traumatic stress.

DOI: 10.4324/9780429317934-3

Learning Theory

Behavior therapy has its roots in experimental psychology. As researchers and behavioral therapists began to study and treat rape victims and Vietnam veterans in the 1970s, they began to draw upon learning theory as an explanation for the fear and anxiety symptoms they were observing. Mowrer's two-factor theory (1947) of classical and operant conditioning was first proposed to account for post-trauma symptoms (Becker et al., 1984; Keane et al., 1985; Kilpatrick et al., 1982, 1985). Classical conditioning was used to explain the high levels of distress and fear that were observed in trauma victims. In this model, the traumatic event is the unconditioned stimulus (UCS), which evokes extreme fear, the unconditioned response (UCR). The trauma (UCS) becomes associated with cues—previously neutral stimuli—which happen to be present during the event, which then become conditioned stimuli (CSs). For example, at the time of an assault, a victim is alone, in the dark, in the parking lot of a grocery store. Thereafter, thinking about or being alone, in the dark, or seeing a parking lot would be CSs that could elicit a conditioned emotional response (CER). A combination of two or three stimuli would prompt a stronger response than any one alone. Thus, anytime these cues are present in the environment, the CSs evoke fear, which now has become the CER. Then, via stimulus generalization and higher order conditioning, other related stimuli are conditioned, as well as the memory and thoughts about the actual event. For example, the person might come to fear all parking lots or even going outside after dark at all.

Normally, in a classical conditioning model, one would expect that the link between the CS and CER would extinguish over time if the original UCS is not repeated. Operant conditioning is used to explain the development of posttraumatic stress disorder (PTSD) avoidance symptoms and maintenance of fear over time despite the fact that the UCS, the traumatic stressor, is no longer present. Because the trauma memory and other cues (CSs) elicit fear and anxiety (CER), these cues are avoided (or escaped from), and the result is a reduction in fear and anxiety. In this manner, avoidance of the CSs is negatively reinforced (the emotions stop with the avoidance, although temporarily), which prevents extinction of the link between the trauma cues (CSs) and anxiety (CER) that would normally be expected without repetition of the trauma itself (UCS). Using the example above, the person who was assaulted may become highly anxious whenever it is dark or they are alone or expected to go out. The victim leaves lights on at night and avoids parking lots. Therefore, they avoid places and activities that feel dangerous whenever possible. They would also attempt to avoid thinking about the assault, because the memory of the event is paired with distress. This, unfortunately, prevents them from learning that these situations and even the memory of the assault are not truly dangerous, and PTSD symptoms may become chronic.

Emotional Processing Theory

Although learning theory accounts for much of the development and maintenance of the fear and avoidance of PTSD, it does not really explain intrusion symptoms, that is, the repetitive memories of the trauma that intrude into the trauma survivor's thoughts in both conscious and unconscious states. Based on Lang's (1977) concept of anxiety development, Foa and Kozak (1986) and Foa et al. (1989) suggested that PTSD emerges due to the development of a fear network in memory that elicits escape and avoidance behavior. Mental fear structures include stimuli (stranger), responses (heart racing), and meaning elements (I am in danger). Anything associated with the trauma may activate the fear structure or schema and subsequent avoidance behavior. The fear network in people with PTSD is thought to be stable and broadly generalized so that it is easily accessed. Chemtob et al. (1988) proposed that these structures are always at least weakly activated in individuals with PTSD and guide their interpretation of events as potentially dangerous.

When reminders of the trauma activate the fear network, the information in the network enters consciousness (intrusive symptoms). Attempts to avoid this activation result in the avoidance symptoms of PTSD. According to emotional processing theory, repetitive and sufficiently prolonged exposure to the traumatic memory in a safe environment will result in habituation (reduction) of the fear and subsequent change in the fear structure. As emotion decreases, individuals with PTSD will begin to modify their meaning elements spontaneously, change their self-statements, and reduce their generalization. However, brief exposures to stimuli will only activate and enhance the avoidance and will actually help maintain the disorder. Through prolonged exposure and habituation during and between therapy sessions, the meaning elements change to reduce the perception of danger, leading to extinction of the feared CS and new learning.

There have been a number of studies that provide support for the idea that people with PTSD have a greater underlying tendency to attend to danger cues (an activated trauma network) than people without PTSD. Rather than relying solely on subjective reports of participants, these experiments demonstrated that people with PTSD have an attentional bias for verbal information that is trauma-related. The most common method for studying attentional bias is a modified Stroop color-naming paradigm (Stroop, 1935). In this task, research participants are asked to name, as fast as they can, the color of print in which words are written, while ignoring the content of the words themselves. The words may be positive, neutral, or negative and are matched for their reading level and commonality. In the case of PTSD studies, the negative words may be generally negative or specifically trauma-related. In studies with Vietnam veterans, rape victims, and disaster survivors, it was found that participants with PTSD were slower to name the colors of words that were trauma-related compared to either control subjects or those who had experienced trauma but did not have PTSD (Cassiday et al., 1992; McNally et al., 1990; Thrasher et al., 1994; Vrana et al., 1995).

Inhibitory Learning

Subsequent to these theories of fear networks, van Minnen and Foa (2006) found that habituation during sessions or between sessions was unnecessary for the reduction of PTSD symptoms and that the fear network remains, at least in part, and particularly in contexts outside of therapy, while competing with new learning. Craske and others (Craske et al., 2008, 2014; Weisman & Rodebaugh, 2018) proposed the enhancement of learning theory with inhibitory learning theory techniques to establish new nonpathological associations and increase the likelihood of their retrieval and use. Inhibitory learning theory was grounded in extinction learning and memory research. Rather than fear reduction during exposure, researchers have experimented with techniques to increase the violation of negative expectancies and to generalize nonthreat associations (Blakey & Abramowitz, 2016; Craske et al., 2014) rather than emphasizing habituation. For example, Blakey and Abramowitz (2019) have focused on dropping safety aids (e.g., having a weapon by the bed) to prevent avoidance of safe but perceived threat and to reactivate fear memories. These authors also discussed maximizing retrieval cues (e.g., using a worksheet with an alternative thought) to increase the retrieval of an inhibitory association (e.g., "I am safe and the doors are locked. Nothing bad has happened in my own home"). Craske et al. (2014) suggested deepened extinction in which multiple fear stimuli are extinguished separately and then combined to enhance extinction.

Cognitive Theories

The cognitive theories are also concerned with information processing, but they focus on the impact of the trauma on a person's belief system and the adjustment that is necessary to reconcile the traumatic event with prior beliefs and expectations. So, while the information processing theories focus more on the structure of cognitive processing and mechanism of fear maintenance, cognitive theories attend more to the content of cognitions; the meaning of trauma; and its impact on beliefs about current and future self, others, and the world. The first and most influential social-cognitive theorist was Horowitz who moved from a more psychodynamic to cognitive processing theory.

Horowitz (1986) proposed that processing is driven by a "completion tendency", the psychological need for new, incompatible information to be integrated with existing beliefs. The completion tendency keeps the trauma information in active memory until the processing is complete and the event is resolved. Horowitz also theorized that there is a basic conflict between the need to resolve and reconcile the event into the person's history and the desire to avoid emotional pain. When the images of the event (flashbacks, nightmares, intrusive recollections), thoughts about the meanings of the trauma, and emotions associated with the trauma become overwhelming, psychological defense mechanisms take over and the person exhibits numbing or avoidance. He suggested a person with PTSD oscillates between phases of intrusion and avoidance and that if successfully processed, the oscillations become less frequent and less intense. Chronic PTSD would mean that the event stays in active memory without becoming fully integrated and still able to stimulate intrusive and avoidant reactions.

Several other researchers and theorists have focused more on the actual content of the cognitions and the idea that basic assumptions about the world and oneself are shattered. Constructivist theories are based on the idea that people actively create their own internal representations of the world (and themselves). New experiences are assigned meaning based on people's personal model of the world (Janoff-Bulman, 1985, 1992; Mahoney & Lyddon, 1988; McCann & Pearlman, 1990). Janoff-Bulman has paid particular attention to three major assumptions that may be shattered in the face of traumatic events: a belief in personal invulnerability ("I am less likely than others to experience misfortune"), the assumption that the world is meaningful (predictable, controllable, and fair), and a perception of oneself as positive or worthy. In research, Janoff-Bulman has found that trauma victims had significantly more negative beliefs in those realms than nonvictims did. She proposed that traumatic events shatter these assumptions and that, as a result, intense psychological crisis ensues. Because prior assumptions are no longer adequate guides for experience, the result is cognitive disintegration and anxiety.

The task for recovery is reconstruction of fundamental schemas (core beliefs) and the establishment of equilibrium. Janoff-Bulman suggested that this process is accomplished by reinterpreting the event to reduce the distance between the prior beliefs and the new beliefs. She pointed out several possible mechanisms such as downward comparison ("It could have been worse. Others have had more devastating traumas"), reevaluating the trauma in terms of benefits or purpose ("This event has made me stronger. I have learned an important lesson"), or self-blame ("It is my fault that it happened. I shouldn't have been there").

Ehlers and Clark (2000) proposed a cognitive model of PTSD. Like the learning theories, it too was focused primarily on threat and fear. Ehlers and Clark recognized the difference between PTSD and the other anxiety disorders it was classified with. The cognitive models of other anxiety disorders focused specifically on fear appraisals to upcoming dangerous events, while clients with PTSD have problems with their memories of the event that carry into the present as a serious current threat ("nowness"). Comparing those with PTSD (versus those with trauma but no PTSD),

Ehlers et al. found that those with PTSD experienced more distress by the intrusions, lack of time perspective (happening now), and lack of context (disconnected from before and afterward). Hackmann et al. (2004) classified main intrusions as warning signals 92% of the time. Ehlers and Clark (2000) proposed that when an autobiographical memory is recalled, it includes both specific information about the event and context information. And because of perceptual priming, they have strong memories of what they encountered before and during the trauma. Those with PTSD fail to update their memories with subsequent information ("I did not die"), but instead the intrusive symptoms continue to trigger cues that the outcome will happen ("I am going to die").

Ehlers and colleagues' research (Ehlers et al., 2002, 2004) has focused on intrusive memories and has found them to be sensory and not about the traumatic event itself but stimuli that occurred just before the traumatic event occurred, thus leading them to conclude that PTSD intrusions are warning signals with the largest emotional impact that continue into the present. In order to test the model that negative appraisals, disjointed trauma memories, and unhelpful coping strategies maintain PTSD, Beierl et al. (2020) conducted a prospective study with a large sample of participants who had been in an emergency department for injuries following violent assault or traffic collision. They followed up at several time points until six months post-injury. Female gender and assault injuries interacted to predict PTSD at six months, but negative appraisals and disjointed memories at one month predicted symptom severity at six months. Cognitive responses during the trauma (mental defeat, giving up during the trauma) were particularly important in leading to negative appraisals and disjointed memories at one month, which had a strong effect on PTSD symptoms at six months. The unhelpful coping strategies, represented by safety behaviors (excessive precautions), responses to intrusions (i.e., thought suppression, rumination, and emotional numbing), and persistent dissociation, played a role in the maintenance of PTSD symptoms. Therefore, this study provided support for the Ehlers et al. cognitive model.

Resick and colleagues (Resick & Schnicke, 1992, 1993; Resick et al., 2024) have argued that post-trauma affect is not limited to fear and that individuals with PTSD may be just as likely to experience a range of other strong emotions, such as shame, anger, or sadness. Some emotions such as fear, anger, or sadness may emanate directly from the trauma ("natural emotions") because the event is interpreted as dangerous and/or abusive, resulting in losses. It is possible that other "manufactured emotions" can result from faulty interpretations made by the trauma survivor. For example, if someone is intentionally attacked by another person, the danger of the situation would lead to a fight-flight response and the attending emotions might be anger or fear. However, if, in the aftermath, the person encountered other people who blamed them for the attack or made other demeaning statements, the person might experience shame or embarrassment. It is possible that a traumatic event might not even produce the fight-flight response because they were betrayed or humiliated and not afraid. These secondary, or manufactured, emotions would have resulted from thoughts and interpretations about the event, rather than the event itself.

Kubany and Manke (1995) have provided other examples of Vietnam veterans who made decisions during combat, often the lesser of two bad choices, only to develop great shame and guilt (and PTSD) afterward because they reappraised their choices as wrong or bad. Litz et al. (2018) assessed over 1,100 active duty military members who were seeking treatment (707 who were randomized into clinical trials and 292 who were subthreshold for PTSD). They categorized the types of traumas the service members experienced during deployment: life-threat self, life-threat others, aftermath of violence, traumatic loss, and moral injury by self or others (violation of moral codes). They found that service members endorsed more non-threat than threat events. In fact, both traumatic loss and moral injury by self were associated with higher levels of reexperiencing than those who experienced a life threat. Because PTSD is more than a fear disorder, it has been moved out of the anxiety disorders, and more attention is being placed on emotions other than fear and fear extinction.

Resick and colleagues (Resick & Schnicke, 1992; Resick et al., 2024) have proposed that information that is congruent with prior beliefs about oneself or the world is assimilated—integrated into previous beliefs—quickly and without effort because the information matches the schema and little attention is needed to incorporate it. If someone started with negative beliefs about themselves and the world, through either prior trauma or environmental information, they would use a new trauma as more proof that their preexisting negative beliefs are true. They are left with very negative beliefs along with consequent emotions.

On the other hand, when something happens that is schema discrepant, individuals must reconcile this event with their beliefs about themselves and the world. Their belief systems, or their schemas, must be altered—accommodated—to incorporate this new information. However, this process is often avoided because of the strong affect associated with the trauma and, frequently, because altering beliefs may in fact leave people feeling more vulnerable to future traumatic events. For example, many people are raised as children to believe that bad things happen to bad people and good things happen to good people. They are not taught the exceptions or probabilities. This just-world belief would need to be altered after something traumatic happened. However, even when victims accept that bad things can happen to them that they aren't responsible for, they may be more anxious about the possibility of future harm. Thus, rather than accommodating their beliefs to incorporate the trauma, trauma survivors may continue to distort (assimilate) the trauma to keep their prior beliefs intact. A typical example of assimilation is for the person to blame themselves instead of the perpetrator in order to continue to believe that bad events are predictable and only occur when one has done something to deserve them.

It may be that cognitive processing does not occur because trauma survivors avoid the strong affect and subsequently never accommodate the information because they do not ever completely, accurately remember what happened or think through what it means (i.e., process the event). Some people are raised believing that emotions are a sign of weakness or that they should be avoided. While people may be able to distract themselves or deflect their affective experience, traumatic events are associated with much greater emotion that cannot be avoided entirely. Individuals with PTSD may have to work hard to shut down their affective response. Moreover, because the information about the traumatic event has not been processed, categorized, and accommodated, the trauma memories continue to emerge during the day as sensory intrusions, flashbacks, or intrusive reminders, or at night in the form of nightmares. The emotional responses and arousal that are part of the trauma memory emerge as well, which triggers further avoidance.

An alternative to assimilation or accommodation is over-accommodation. In this case, trauma survivors alter their belief structure to the extreme in an attempt to prevent future traumas. These overgeneralized beliefs may take the form of extreme distrust and negative regard for self and others. Prior traumatic events or negative preexisting beliefs would contribute to "the evidence" that these extreme statements are true. For example, a rape victim may believe that no one can be trusted or that she is damaged and worthless because of the rape. A veteran might state that anyone who is associated with the government (even a therapist at a Veterans Administration hospital) is bad or is trying to "mess" with him. These over-accommodated beliefs interfere with the natural emotions that emanated from the event (e.g., fear, sadness) and therefore prevent appropriate processing of the emotions and beliefs. Furthermore, overgeneralized negative statements can produce a different set of emotions that might not have originally been associated with the event (e.g., shame, guilt).

Given this cognitive model, affective expression is needed, not for habituation but in order for the trauma memory to be processed fully into more balanced thinking. It is assumed that the natural affect, once accessed, will dissipate rather quickly (except perhaps grief), and that the work of accommodating the memory with schemas can begin. Once faulty beliefs regarding the event (erroneous self-blame, guilt) and over-accommodated beliefs about oneself and the world (e.g. safety, trust, control, esteem, intimacy) are examined, then the secondary emotions will also diminish along with the intrusive reminders. There have been several studies that have showed cognitive change precedes change in PTSD symptoms (e.g., Schumm et al., 2015).

Dual Representation Theory

Viewing PTSD as a disorder of memory due to the frequent involuntary images as flashbacks, nightmares, or intrusive images, Brewin et al. (1996) proposed a dual representation theory. Brewin et al. suggested that the concept of a unitary memory system is unable to account for the full range of phenomena that have been detailed in research and clinical observations. Based on prior research, they proposed that sensory input is subject to both conscious and nonconscious processing. The aspects of the traumatic event that are consciously attended to can be deliberately retrieved and are termed "verbally accessible memories". Because attention may be narrowed by the presence of an imminent threat (such as a gun), other aspects of the event are apprehended only briefly and are stored as images (situationally accessible memories). Brewin et al. (2010) revised the theory and terminology based on the inclusion of what had been learned in the meantime about intrusions in other disorders and brain functioning (which will be covered more in Chapter 4).

The updated research and theory on memory focuses on perceptual and episodic memory, particularly as they relate to intrusive symptoms of PTSD. Brewin and his colleagues (Brewin, 2010, 2014; Bisby et al., 2020) have proposed that there are two memory systems: First, there is ordinary episodic memory in which the different elements of an event are integrated by the hippocampus into a coherent, contextualized memory. The second memory system allows individual perceptual features to become associated with emotional arousal after experiences such as traumatic events. Negative emotions activate the amygdala but reduce hippocampal activity.

Bisby et al. (2020) reviewed studies with both animals and humans pertaining to this model. In PTSD, flashbacks and intrusive images are involuntary sensory memories (S-reps) that are highly distressing, without much context, and with a sense of occurring here and now. They are contrasted with verbal autobiographical memories (C-reps). During a trauma, the S-reps (the perceptual memories) are encoded in great sensory detail, while the C-reps (the contextualized episodic memories) are weakened as are the connections between C-reps and S-reps. C-reps are retrieved intentionally when the person talks or thinks about the traumatic event; however, verbal voluntary recall of the event may be fragmented and disorganized. Because C-reps are conscious, language-based memories, they can also be modified with alternative points of view.

Transdiagnostic Model

The transdiagnostic model of treatment has become increasingly popular over the past decade in an attempt to treat comorbid disorders simultaneously. The transdiagnostic model comes from the observation that many mood and anxiety disorders are not only comorbid but have some underlying traits in common. The argument is that disorders may have some unique features, but they often have more in common with each other than differences. PTSD is a disorder with very high comorbidity with other disorders. For example, most studies find at least 50% comorbidity with depression. Some of the transdiagnostic variables that have been examined in PTSD are low distress tolerance (Boffa et al., 2018) and sleep disturbance (Britton et al., 2019). Gallagher (2017) summarized several mechanisms across diagnoses: hope, neuroticism (temperamental disposition to experience and respond to negative emotions), emotion regulation, cognitions and cognitive reappraisal, and anxiety sensitivity (fear of anxiety and related bodily sensations). Catastrophic thinking has also been identified as a transdiagnostic process across disorders (Gellatly & Beck, 2016). Hernández-Posadas et al. (2023) conducted a meta-analysis finding that rumination and emotional dysregulation were robust predictors of PTSD and depression in cross-sectional and longitudinal studies.

Despite the growing popularity of the approach and particularly transdiagnostic therapies, research on the model and underlying theory has been somewhat scant. One theory that moves beyond just a description of symptom overlap is a memory-based transdiagnostic theory of emotional disorders (Cohen & Kahana, 2022). They cite Brewin's work on PTSD and depression as both having high rates of vivid, intrusive memories and that patients recall negative events more readily than positive events. Cohen and Kahana refer to a retrieved-context theory that proposes a unitary memory system and not two. Their theory and research propose that emotional intensity, repetition, and rehearsal strengthen how accessible the memory becomes such that it spontaneously activates. While dual representation theory proposes that trauma memories in PTSD have unique properties that differ from those found in other disorders, the retrieved-context theory proposes one memory system of mood congruent recall that would be transdiagnostic.

Summary

At this point in time, predominant theories of PTSD focus on learning theory including the addition of inhibitory learning, cognitive theory with an emphasis on content of cognitions, or memory processes implicated in the intrusive symptoms. All have research to support them, and they may all comprise components of an overall understanding of why some people recover from traumatic events, while others go on to develop the chronic and complicated symptoms of PTSD. This may also explain why using very different approaches, the majority of people benefit from treatment.

References

Becker, J. V., Skinner, L. J., Abel, G. G., Axelrod, R., & Cichon, J. (1984). Sexual problems of sexual assault survivors. *Women and Health, 9*, 5–20.

Beierl, E. T., Böllinghaus, I., Clark, D. M., Glucksman, E., & Ehlers, A. (2020). Cognitive paths from trauma to posttraumatic stress disorder: A prospective study of Ehlers and Clark's model in survivors of assaults or road traffic collisions. *Psychological Medicine, 50*, 2172–2181.

Bisby, J. A., Burgess, N., & Brewin, C. R. (2020). Reduced memory coherence for negative events and its relationship to posttraumatic stress disorder. *Current Directions in Psychological Science, 29*, 267–272.

Blakey, S. M., & Abramowitz, J. S. (2016). The effects of safety behaviors during exposure therapy for anxiety: Critical analysis from an inhibitory learning perspective. *Clinical Psychology Review, 49*, 1–15.

Blakey, S. M., & Abramowitz, J. S. (2019). Dropping safety aids and maximizing retrieval cues: Two keys to optimizing inhibitory learning during exposure therapy. *Cognitive and Behavioral Practice, 26*, 166–175.

Boffa, J. W., Short, N. A., Gibby, B. A., Stentz, L. A., & Schmidt N. B. (2018). Distress tolerance as a mechanism of PTSD symptom change: Evidence for mediation in a treatment-seeking sample. *Psychiatry Research, 267*, 400–408.

Brewin, C. R. (2014). Episodic memory, perceptual memory, and their interaction: Foundations for a theory of posttraumatic stress disorder. *Psychological Bulletin, 140*, 69–97.

Brewin, C. R., Dalgleish, T., & Joseph, S. (1996). A dual representation theory of posttraumatic stress disorder. *Psychological Review, 103*, 670–686.

Brewin, C. R., Gregory, J. D., Lipton, M., & Burgess, N. (2010). Intrusive images in psychological disorders: Characteristics, neural mechanisms, and treatment implications. *Psychological Review, 117*, 210–232.

Britton, P. C., McKinney, J. M., Bishop, T. M., Pigeon, W. R., & Hirsch, J. K. (2019) Insomnia and risk for suicidal behavior: A test of a mechanistic transdiagnostic model in veterans. *Journal of Affective Disorders, 245*, 412–418.

Cassiday, K. L., McNally, R. J., & Zeitlin, S. B. (1992). Cognitive processing of trauma cues in rape victims with post- traumatic stress disorder. *Cognitive Therapy and Research, 16*, 283–295.

Chemtob, C., Roitblat, H. L., Hamada, R. S., Carlson, J. G., & Twentyman, C. T. (1988). A cognitive action theory of post-traumatic stress disorder. *Journal of Anxiety Disorders, 2*, 253–275.

Cohen, R. T., & Kahana, M. J. (2022) A memory based theory of emotional disorders. *Psychological Review, 129*, 742–776.

Craske, M. G., Kircanski, K., Zelikowsky, M., Mystkowski, J., Chowdhury, N., & Baker, A. (2008). Optimizing inhibitory learning during exposure therapy. *Behaviour Research and Therapy, 46*, 5–27.

Craske, M. G., Treanor, M., Conway, C. C., Zbozinek, T., & Vervliet, B. (2014). Maximizing exposure therapy: An inhibitory learning approach. *Behaviour Research and Therapy, 58*, 10–23.

Ehlers, A., & Clark, D. M. (2000). A cognitive model of posttraumatic stress disorder. *Behaviour Research and Therapy, 38*, 319–345.

Ehlers, A., Hackmann, A., & Michael, T. (2004). Intrusive re-experiencing in post-traumatic stress disorder: Phenominology, theory, and therapy. *Memory, 12*, 403–415.

Ehlers, A., Hackmann, A., Steil, R., Clohessy, S., Wenninger, K., & Winter, H. (2002). The nature of intrusive memories after trauma: The warning signal hypothesis. *Behaviour Research and Therapy, 40*, 1021–1028.

Foa, E. B., & Kozak, M. J. (1986). Emotional processing of fear: Exposure to corrective information. *Psychological Bulletin, 99*, 20–35.

Foa, E. B., Steketee, G., & Rothbaum, B. O. (1989). Behavioral/cognitive conceptualizations of post-traumatic stress disorder. *Behavior Therapy, 20*, 155–176.

Gallagher, M. W. (2017). Transdiagnostic mechanisms of change and cognitive-behavioral treatments for PTSD. *Current Opinion in Psychology, 14*, 90–95.

Gellatly, R., & Beck, A. T. (2016). Catastrophic thinking: A transdiagnostic process across psychiatric disorders. *Cognitive Therapy Research, 40*, 441–452.

Hackmann, A., Ehlers, A., Speckens, A., & Clark, D. M. (2004). Characteristics and content of intrusive memories in PTSD and their changes with treatment. *Journal of Traumatic Stress, 17*, 231–240.

Hernández-Posadas, A., Lommen, M. J. J., de la Rosa Gómez, A., Bouman, T. K., Mancilla-Díaz, J. M., & del Palacio González, A. (2023). Transdiagnostic factors in symptoms of depression and post-traumatic stress: A systematic review, *Current Psychology*, published online, https://doi.org/10.1007/s12144-023-04792-x

Horowitz, M. (1986). *Stress response syndromes* (2nd ed.). New York: Aronson.

Janoff-Bulman, R. (1985). The aftermath of victimization: Rebuilding shattered assumptions. In C. R. Figley (Ed.), *Trauma and its wake: The study and treatment of post-traumatic stress disorder* (pp. 15–35). New York: Brunner/Mazel.

Janoff-Bulman, R. (1992). *Shattered assumptions: Towards a new psychology of trauma.* New York: The Free Press.

Keane, T. M., Zimering, R. T., & Caddell, R. T. (1985). A behavioral formulation of PTSD in Vietnam veterans. *The Behavior Therapist, 8*, 9–12.

Kilpatrick, D. G., Veronen, L. J., & Best, C. L. (1985). Factors predicting psychological distress among rape victims. In C. R. Figley (Ed.), *Trauma and its wake* (pp. 113–141). New York: Brunner/Mazel.

Kilpatrick, D. G., Veronen, L, J., & Resick, P. A. (1982). Psychological sequelae to rape: Assesssment and treatment strategies. In D. M. Dolays, R. L. Meredith & A. R. Ciminero (Eds.), *Behavioral medicine: assessment and treatment strategies* (pp. 473–497). New York: Plenum Press.

Kubany, E. S., & Manke, F. P. (1995). Cognitive therapy for trauma-related guilt: Conceptual bases and treatment outlines. *Cognitive and Behavioral Practice, 2*, 27–61.

Lang, P. J. (1977). Imagery in therapy: An information processing analysis of fear. *Behavior Therapy, 8*, 862–886.

Litz, B. T., Contractor, A. A., Rhodes, C., Dondanville, K. A., Jordan, A. H., Resick, P. A., Foa, E. B., Young-McCaughan, S., Mintz, J., Yarvis, J. S., & Peterson, A. L. (2018). Distinct trauma types in military service members seeking treatment for posttraumatic stress disorder. *Journal of Traumatic Stress, 31*, 286–295.

Mahoney, M., & Lyddon, W. (1988). Recent developments in cognitive approaches to counseling and psychotherapy. *Counseling Psychologist, 16*, 190–234.

McCann, I. L., & Pearlman, L. A. (1990). *Psychological trauma and the adult survivor: Theory, therapy, and transformation.* New York: Brunner/Mazel.

McNally, R. J., Kaspi, S. P., Reiman, B. C., & Zeitlin, S. B. (1990). Selective processing of threat cues in post-traumatic stress disorder. *Journal of Abnormal Psychology, 99*, 398–402.

Mower, O. H. (1947). On the dual nature of learning: A reinterpretation of "conditioning" and "problem solving." *Harvard Educational Review, 17*, 102–148.

Resick, P. A., Monson, C. M., & Chard, K. M. (2024). *Cognitive processing therapy for PTSD: A comprehensive therapist manual, Second Edition.* New York: Guilford.

Resick, P. A., & Schnicke, M. K. (1992). Cognitive processing therapy for sexual assault victims. *Journal of Consulting and Clinical Psychology, 60*, 748–756.

Resick, P. A., & Schnicke, M. K. (1993). *Cognitive processing therapy for rape victims: A treatment manual.* Newbury Park, CA: Sage Publications.

Schumm, J. A., Dickstein, B. D., Walter, K. H., Owens, G. P., & Chard, K. M. (2015). Changes in posttraumatic cognitions predict changes in posttraumatic stress disorder symptoms during cognitive processing therapy. *Journal of Consulting and Clinical Psychology, 83*, 1161–1166.

Stroop, J. R. (1935). Studies of interference in serial verbal reaction. *Journal of Experimental Psychology, 18*, 643–662.

Thrasher, S. M., Dangleish, T., & Yule, W. (1994). Information processing in post-traumatic stress disorder. *Behavior Research and Therapy, 32*, 247–254.

Van Minnen, A., & Foa, E. B. (2006). The effect of imaginal exposure length on outcome of treatment for PTSD. *Journal of Traumatic Stress, 19*, 427–438.

Vrana, S. R., Roodman, A., & Beckham, J. C. (1995). Selective processing of trauma-relevant words in posttraumatic stress disorder. *Journal of Anxiety Disorders, 9*, 515–530.

Weisman, J. S., & Rodebaugh, T. L. (2018). Exposure therapy augmentation: A review and extension of techniques informed by an inhibitory learning approach. *Clinical Psychology Review, 59*, 41–51.

4

The Biology of PTSD

Research on psychophysiology, neurochemistry, genetics, relevant brain structures, brain networks, and whole brain studies of posttraumatic stress disorder (PTSD) have exploded in the past two decades. PTSD is affected by many systems and affects them in turn. This chapter will just skim the surface of all that has been studied but should provide an overview of the field. Because the field of PTSD began with the classification of PTSD as an anxiety disorder, the initial emphasis was on fear circuitry. More recently, studies have moved to broader definitions of symptoms including affect regulation more generally and the role of cognition.

Psychophysiology

The first studies that examined the biology of PTSD focused on the fear response with physiological studies of heart rate, skin conductance, or facial electromyogram (EMG; a measure of muscular response) and have continued for decades. The study of psychophysiological reactivity is quite old in fact. Meakins and Wilson (1918) found that World War I veterans with "shell-shock" had greater increases in respiration and heart rate upon exposure to sulfuric flames and sounds of gunfire than healthy comparison subjects. Also in 1918, Fraser and Wilson found that when war veterans were administered epinephrine, they had exaggerated psychophysiological arousal. In 1941, Abraham Kardiner labeled traumatic stress "physioneurosis", recognizing the connection between physiological and psychological reactions to traumatic stress.

The typical research design since the 1980s has been to examine the psychophysiological reactivity during a resting baseline period and then to examine reactions to neutral, generic stressful, or trauma-related stimuli. The generic stressful stimuli may

DOI: 10.4324/9780429317934-4

be stressors such as mental arithmetic or a public speaking fear script, which most people react to with increased arousal. Trauma-related stimuli may include sounds or visual images such as slides or film depicting combat accompanied by recorded combat noises; they may be generic trauma scripts that are presented to all the research participants, or they may be individualized scripts, which have proven to be the most effective in eliciting a response.

When individualized scripts are used, the researcher meets with the participant in advance and develops a short vignette that describes the actual event the participant experienced, including sensory details, emotions, and physical reactions. Typically, the participant is presented with the script orally, and then they are instructed to imagine the scene as vividly as possible. Most studies found that about two-thirds of participants with and without PTSD were correctly classified, with those with PTSD showing elevated psychophysiological responses. After several small studies of psychophysiological assessment (e.g., Blanchard et al., 1996; Orr et al., 1998, 2004 for review; Pitman et al., 1987, 1990), there was a large multisite study (Keane et al., 1998) that found the same with 654 participants with current PTSD, 154 with lifetime PTSD, and 340 participants without PTSD. They also found that the majority of people with PTSD showed physiological arousal.

Psychophysiological assessment was advocated for diagnosis, but it is not universal because PTSD is not always dominated by fear (Ramage et al., 2016). Some people with PTSD have a response that is more cognitive and may involve guilt and shame rather than fear. Pitman et al. (2012) suggested that pretreatment psychophysiological assessment could be used to guide treatment selection. They posited that those who had higher psychophysiological reactivity to trauma cues might benefit more to exposure-based therapies. One study that has looked at psychophysiological functioning collapsed an exposure therapy (prolonged exposure) with a more cognitive therapy (cognitive processing therapy) to examine treatment responders and nonresponders (Griffin et al., 2012). They found that startle response to loud tones did decrease among the treatment responders but did not have a large enough sample to determine if it worked better for one treatment or the other.

Neuroendocrine Studies

The lion's share of studies on endocrine functioning in PTSD has focused on cortisol, the stress hormone. There have been many studies demonstrating that people who experienced traumatic events had alterations in the hypothalamic-pituitary-adrenal (HPA) axis. When someone experiences a stressful event, the HPA axis is activated, and cortisol is released into the bloodstream, which triggers the sympathetic nervous system and the fight-flight-freeze response. Cortisol is the product of this activation and plays an important role in bringing the body back to normal (see Olff & van Zuiden, 2017, for review). The effects of cortisol during stress are enacted by binding to glucocorticoid receptors, which then affect immunosuppression, higher energy metabolism, and negative feedback of the HPA axis, all needed during stress for the fight-flight response. One does not need immune responses if one is in imminent danger and the HPA axis needs to stay activated. Once the danger is passed, normal immune function returns.

Because HPA axis activation is intended to be a short-term response to threat, it was hypothesized that, in people with PTSD, there would be dysregulation and that they would show continuously elevated cortisol, much like is found in depression. It was hoped to be a biological marker of PTSD that could be easily assessed in urine, blood, saliva, and even hair. However, counter to expectations, research showed that people with PTSD had low morning cortisol levels and were also lower in the evening than trauma-exposed controls without PTSD (Morris et al., 2012). This appears to be the case because PTSD symptoms like flashbacks and fear-inducing triggers that generalize over time result in increased glucocorticoid receptors to receive the cortisol (Yehuda et al., 1991). In keeping with the lower cortisol, the immune system is activated, which leads to inflammation. This cortisol response is not observed in everyone with PTSD, but, as is explained throughout this chapter and book, PTSD is a heterogeneous disorder and not everyone has a fear response during or after their traumas. In those with this suppressed cortisol response, there are correlated health risks including cardiovascular disease, rheumatoid arthritis, and dementia.

One question that was examined was whether people have pretrauma neuroendocrine risk factors for PTSD. Olff and van Zuiden (2017) reported on several studies of military or police who showed low pretrauma cortisol levels, low cortisol stress reactivity, or high pretrauma glucocorticoid receptors among those who subsequently developed PTSD.

Although this section has focused on cortisol and receptors, there have been dozens of other neuroendocrine systems that have been studied in PTSD as the greater complexity of the disorder's effects on the brain and body has been understood. It is beyond the scope of this brief chapter on the biology of PTSD to describe all of them. For those with greater interest in the topic, Rasmusson et al. (2021) will be a good resource.

Genetics

Because the rate of exposure to traumatic events over the course of a lifetime is very high, but the rate of those people who have resulting PTSD is relatively low, there has been an effort to determine if genetics plays a role in susceptibility to PTSD.

According to a Pitman et al. (2012) review, genetics account for 30–72% of vulnerability to PTSD. Prior to actually studying genes, there were many studies to determine if PTSD runs in families. Leen-Feldner et al. (2013) reviewed over 100 studies of offspring of parents with posttraumatic stress. While there is a relationship between parents and children in the development of PTSD, the problem is that genetics are entangled with the environment. In order to disentangle the effects of genetic and environmental factors, research moved to twin studies, assuming a shared environment (or being able to account for it better). These studies compared fraternal (dizygotic) twins with identical (monozygotic) twins because dizygotic twins share 50% of genes, while monozygotic twins share 100% of genes. In the 1980s, the Department of Veterans Affairs set up a Vietnam Era Twin Registry of middle-aged Vietnam veterans who were measured over time to examine the genetics of various illnesses (Goldberg, 2002). True et al. (1993) conducted an examination of 4,042 male monozygotic and dizygotic veterans' genetic and environmental contributions to posttraumatic stress symptoms and unique environment. They found significant genetic influences on symptoms even after adjusting for combat exposure. The correlations of various symptoms were much lower for dizygotic twins than for monozygotic twins even after taking into account combat exposure.

Overall, twin studies with various populations have found that exposure to trauma is influenced by genetic factors; the heritability for exposure in civilian samples is 38% and 35–47% in combat exposure (Bustamante et al., 2021; Sheerin et al., 2017; Voisey et al., 2014). Furthermore, genetic influences explain 30% of PTSD among male Vietnam veterans but 72% among young women. These studies found that genetics play a role in other disorders aside from PTSD and especially a shared effect between PTSD and depression, generalized anxiety disorder, panic disorder, and substance use.

The next step in studying genetics was to select candidate genes to see if they were related to PTSD. The selection of genes to study was based on the knowledge of the biology of PTSD at the time. As many as 100 studies have been conducted with dozens of different genes examined. Unfortunately, the samples were typically small and not replicated. There appear to be more complex relationships between genes and environment that need to be explored.

Taking a more objective (agnostic) approach, there have been genome-wide association studies (GWAS) that examine the entire genome with very large samples to see if any patterns emerged. In order to conduct such studies, consortia across centers have been created. Very large samples are required to find small effects, much smaller than the twin studies have indicated. However, they have found genes that link to reexperencing symptoms, arousal, memory, immune function, and inflammation (Bustamante et al., 2021).

Genetics is not a one-way street. PTSD can change gene expression, and prior trauma can affect genetics leading to risk for future PTSD. This has led to epigenetic studies. DNA methylation is one of the major ways that genetic functions are changed. DNA methylation is an epigenetic mechanism in the body in which a small molecule called a methyl group is added to DNA, proteins, or other molecules, which can act to turn on or off a gene. Epigenetic studies can be used with either candidate genes or GWAS. It is logical with PTSD to study the effects of trauma and stress on genetics. Studies have found expression within genes to be involved in the HPA axis and immune functioning between those with and without PTSD (Sheerin et al., 2017).

Brain Structures and PTSD

Harnett et al. (2020) provide a helpful review of structures of the brain related to PTSD. Understanding of the function of brain structures came first from lesion studies, intentional in rodents and with accidents or diseases in humans. Then with the advent of positron emission tomography (PET) scans, computerized tomography (CT) scans, computerized axial tomography (CAT) scans, and functional magnetic resonance imaging (MRI), research exploded. The first two brain structures to receive attention were the hippocampus and amygdala. The hippocampus and amygdala form one of the circuits in the limbic system, which affects behaviors related to self-preservation, learning and memory, and emotion. The hippocampus receives information from all regions of the sensory association cortex, motor association cortex, and amygdala, and appears to have a coordinating or mapping function that puts information into context. The hippocampus is also involved in short-term memory, such that memories are held temporarily, after which they are either stored in long-term memory or forgotten.

The hippocampus is believed to be essential in declarative memory. Declarative memory is memory that a person can state in words, the retelling of things the person knows or events previously experienced (as opposed to procedural memory, which reflects motor skills). It appears that the hippocampus is involved in tying together the different perceptions involved in an event and plays a role in fear learning and extinction. Therefore, the hippocampus enables relational learning between stimuli. Many studies, usually with small samples, have shown through brain imaging that in PTSD there is a smaller hippocampal volume, although others have not. In order to examine this further, a large consortium (Logue et al., 2017) of 16 groups from five countries studied PTSD patients and control groups with various levels of trauma exposure (in total, data from 1,868 subjects, including 794 PTSD patients and 1,074 control subjects). They found significantly smaller hippocampal volume among those with PTSD. Although there has been some question as to whether the hippocampus shrinks as a result of PTSD or people with a smaller hippocampus are more likely to develop PTSD, there appears to be a connection between hippocampal volume and PTSD.

The amygdala, also receiving a lot of early attention among those conducting imaging studies, is located in the temporal lobes. It is the most important part of the brain for the expression of emotional responses that are provoked by negative stimuli and has a strong connection with the hippocampus in acquiring conditioned fear. The amygdala receives input directly from the sensory cortex. The amygdala is important in learning the emotional significance of external events, particularly social actions, and is an important component of the fight-flight response. Unlike the volume studies, the amygdala attracted attention because it was shown to be activated in imaging studies when participants were shown fear pictures or listened to trauma scripts. It has been referred to as a salience or threat detector (Andrewes & Jenkins, 2019) and affects autonomic preparation for fight, flight, or freeze responses. The amygdala, simply speaking, is part of a feedback loop with the executive portion of the brain, the prefrontal cortex (PFC) and its component parts, in what Andrewes and Jenkins (2019) referred to as a dual inhibition model. When the PFC is activated, it serves to regulate emotions; it inhibits the amygdala and brings it back to a resting state. This is what happens under normal circumstances when someone has a sudden threat. However, in people with PTSD, the picture is somewhat different. The amygdala becomes increasingly activated (especially with generalization of trauma cues), and the PFC fails to inhibit the activity, leading to affect dysregulation. Also, in PTSD, the usual strong connections between the PFC and the hippocampus are reduced, resulting in a failure to extinguish learned fear and provide a rational memory perspective (impaired ability to distinguish safe from dangerous contexts).

Aside from the fight-flight response, there are other areas that pertain to cognition in PTSD. Not all PTSD is explained by fear conditioning. The components of the PFC are also associated with executive functions. In a study with treatment seeking active duty service members with PTSD who were randomized to either cognitive processing therapy or present centered therapy, imaging demonstrated that with cognitive processing therapy, there was an increase in executive functioning from pre- to posttreatment (Abdallah et al., 2019).

The precuneus is a hub with connections to other brain areas with autobiographical and self-reflective functions. In an active duty military treatment seeking sample, participants were given PET scans (Ramage et al., 2016). They were compared to combat controls and civilian controls. The primary traumas were classified as danger (direct threat to self or others) or nondanger (aftermath of violence such as body handling, witnessing or learning about death of friend/family member, moral injury by self or others). Those who experienced a danger trauma reacted as expected with greater amygdala activation. Those who had PTSD from non-danger traumas had a lower response identical to the combat controls or civilian controls. On the other hand, the non-danger PTSD group had a stronger response in the left precuneus, while the danger group, combat controls, and civilian controls did not differ from each other. Philippi et al. (2020) studied resting-state imaging in women with PTSD and found that the left precuneus was associated with rumination.

Compared to many other brain structures, the cerebellum had largely been ignored in PTSD research because it has long been considered to be only concerned with motor functions. Because of the development of newer brain scan technology that examines connections between structures across the whole brain instead of just those that were hypothesized to be involved in PTSD, new findings have emerged. The cerebellum sends and receives information to non-motor cortical areas, including prefrontal structures associated with higher cognitive functions. In both adults and adolescents with PTSD, lower cerebellum volume is correlated with PTSD symptoms. Lesions to the cerebellum can result in anxiety, aggression, irritability, and distractibility, all symptoms associated with PTSD (Holmes et al., 2018).

Brain Networks

There is increasing evidence that brain structures are organized beyond particular circuits that had been previously identified such as fear circuitry (Averall et al., 2021). Once functional MRI became more sophisticated, allowing for whole brain scans, there was what Menon (2011) labeled a paradigm shift in looking at dysfunctional brain functioning over time tied to specific psychiatric disorders. The examination of brain networks, defined as collections of brain regions that are linked, focused on three core networks, called the triple-network model, consisting of the central executive network (CEN), the default mode network (DMN), and the salience network (SN; Averall et al., 2021).

The CEN is composed of parts of the PFC, the middle frontal gyrus, and the precuneus. If the CEN is disrupted, there may be problems with goal-directed activity and memory, and in PTSD there is weaker connectivity within the CEN, leading to loss of top-down regulation and cognitive deficits. The DMN is comprised of the posterior cingulate cortex, the medial PFC, and the medial temporal lobe (including the hippocampus). The DMN focuses on self-referential, introspection, and autobiographical memory, active during rest. This resting-state functional connection is decreased in PTSD and associated with dissociation, avoidance, and intrusive symptoms. The SN components identified so far are the amygdala, the insula, and the dorsal anterior cingulate cortex. The SN is involved in the detection of salient (relevant) internal and external stimuli. In PTSD there is heightened threat detection and impaired modulation. In a review of network research in PTSD (Akiki et al., 2018), it was noted that there may be a weakly connected and hypoactive CEN and DMN that is destabilized by an overactive and hyperconnected SN. Therefore, there is a low threshold for perceived salience and ineffective CEN and DMN modulation.

Dissociation

Although dissociative disorders can be separate from PTSD, in the DSM-5 it was decided that there was enough evidence to include a dissociative subtype with the diagnosis of PTSD. This resulted from a consistent finding across epidemiological, physiological, brain imaging, and even treatment research that there is a minority but significant number of people with PTSD who respond differently than the majority without dissociation. First, the definition of dissociation is that there is a disruption or discontinuity of consciousness. It involves subjective detachment from the traumatic memory and can lead to fragmentation of the memory. It can occur during traumatic events ("peritraumatic dissociation") in which both fight and flight responses fail and may prove to be the coping response of last resort (e.g., child sexual abuse or torture). Dissociation can also become an ongoing response when trauma has become repeated and when triggers generalize into everyday life. There are generally two types of dissociation that are found in the dissociative subtype: depersonalization (detached from one's body and mind, feeling unreal) and derealization (feeling detached from surroundings, as if in a dream). Other dissociative symptoms such as flashbacks and amnesia are common in PTSD, so the focus on the subtype is on depersonalization and derealization which are not already part of the PTSD symptoms.

Griffin et al. (1997) studied psychophysiological reactivity among recent rape victims using a somewhat different methodology than prior studies that used script-driven imagery. Rather than listening to scripts, participants were asked to talk for five minutes on a neutral recall topic or to describe their rapes. These neutral and trauma phases were interspersed with baseline conditions. Rather than looking at the PTSD group as a whole, Griffin et al. examined skin conductance and heart rate with regard to peritraumatic dissociation (PD)—the extent to which someone dissociated during the traumatic event. They found a smaller group (19%) of highly dissociative women who responded in a very different manner than the other women with PTSD. While the skin conductance and heart rate of those with low PD scores increased as expected while they were talking about the rape, those with high PD scores showed a decrease in the physiological measures. When they examined the participants' subjective distress during each of the phases, the high PD group reported the same level of distress as the low PD group. Therefore, while they were experiencing distress, their physiological responses were suppressed. Griffin et al. (1997) speculated that there may be a dissociative subtype of PTSD that responds quite differently than the more phobic type of PTSD. This might explain why some studies have found a proportion of PTSD nonresponders in physiological studies.

In descriptive studies of PTSD in which the factors of PTSD and dissociation are determined, several veteran and civilian studies found similar findings. Wolf and colleagues (2012a, 2012b) conducted analyses on groups of veterans and found three types: one with low PTSD, one with high PTSD, and a smaller but distinct group with high PTSD and dissociative symptoms. The dissociative groups made up 12–15% of the sample, although one study found that a sample of women contained 30% with the dissociative subtype. Steuwe et al. (2012) examined a civilian sample of people who had PTSD predominantly from childhood abuse and found that 25% fell into the group with high dissociation (measuring depersonalization and derealization). The biggest study, with over 25,000 participants from 16 countries from the World Health Organization World Mental Health Survey, showed that 14% of the sample experienced depersonalization or derealization (Stein et al., 2013).

Aside from the drop in skin conductance and heart rate found in the Griffin et al. (1997) study, Lanius et al. (2002) found matching brain imaging patterns and nonresponse on heart rate to script-driven imagery. While the majority of people with PTSD show undermodulation of affect with an increase in amygdala responding and a correlated decrease in activity in the PFC, as described above, the dissociative subtype shows overmodulation, just the opposite. Those with high dissociation when a level of anxiety is reached activate the medial PFC, which inhibits the limbic system including the amygdala. In other words, along with the perceptions of derealization and depersonalization, there is a lack of reactivity. They also show hyperinhibition in response to painful stimuli (see Lanius et al., 2012, 2014, for reviews).

Summary

Biological studies using physiological and neuroendocrine measures to genetics and brain imaging have all found strong evidence for PTSD to have effects on the brain and functioning that help explain the symptoms of PTSD. The field is growing constantly, and brain networks appear to be a particularly exciting avenue to tie together many of the varied symptoms of PTSD. Dissociative responses have been shown to be quite different with regard to overmodulation rather than the typical PTSD response of undermodulation of emotions in PTSD. These physiological and imaging results have helped confirm the presence of a dissociative subtype of PTSD.

References

Abdallah, C. G., Averill, C. L., Ramage, A. E., Averill, L. A., Alkin, E., Nemati, S., Krystal, J. H., Roache, J. D., Resick, P. A., Young-McCaughan, S., Peterson, A. L., & Fox, P. T., and the STRONG STAR Consortium. (2019). Reduced salience and enhanced central executive connectivity following PTSD treatment. *Chronic Stress, 3*, 1–10.

Akiki, T. J., Averill, C. L., & Abdallah, C. G. (2018). A network-based neurobiological model of PTSD: Evidence from structural and functional neuroimaging studies. *Current Psychiatry Reports, 19*, 81.

Andrewes, N. G., & Jenkins, L. M. (2019). The role of the amygdala and the ventromedial prefrontal cortex in emotional regulation: Implications for post-traumatic stress disorder. *Neuropsychology Review, 29*, 220–243.

Averall, L. A., Averill, C. L., Akiki, T. J., & Abdallah C. G. (2021). Examining neurocircuitry and neuroplasticity in PTSD. In M. J. Friedman, P. P. Schnurr & T. M. Keane (Eds.), *Handbook of PTSD: Science and practice* (3rd ed., pp. 152–167). New York: Guilford Press.

Blanchard, E. B., Hickling, E. J., Buckley, T. C., Taylor, A. E., Vollmer, A., & Loos, W. R. (1996). Psychophysiology of posttraumatic stress disorder related to motor vehicle accidents: Replication and extension. *Journal of Consulting and Clinical Psychology, 64*, 742–751.

Bustamante, D., Bountress, K., Sheerin, C., Koenen, K. C., Guffanti, G., Yan, L., Haloossim, M., Uddin, M., Nugent, N., & Amstadter, A. B. (2021). Chapter 11: Genetics of PTSD. In M. J. Friedman, P. P. Schnurr & T. M. Keane (Eds.), *Handbook of PTSD: Science and practice* (3rd ed., pp. 192–210). New York: Guilford Press.

Fraser, F., & Wilson, E. M. (1918). The sympathetic nervous system and the "irritable heart of soldiers." *British Medical Journal, 2*, 27–29.

Goldberg, J., Curran, B., Vitek, M. E., Henderson, W. G., & Boyko, E. J. (2002). The Vietnam era twin registry. *Twin Research and Human Genetics, 5*, 476–481.

Griffin, M. G., Resick, P. A., & Galovski, T. E. (2012). Does physiologic response to loud tones change following cognitive-behavioral treatment for posttraumatic stress disorder? *Journal of Traumatic Stress, 25*, 25–32.

Griffin, M. G., Resick, P. A., & Mechanic, M. B. (1997). Objective assessment of peritraumatic dissociation: Psychophysiological indicators. *American Journal of Psychiatry, 154*, 1081–1088.

Harnett, N. G., Goodman, A. M., & Knight, D. C. (2020). PTSD-related neuroimaging abnormalities in brain function, structure, and biochemistry. *Experimental Neurology, 330*, 113331.

Holmes, S. E., Scheinost, D., DellaGioia, N., Davis, M. T., Matuskey, D., Pietrzak, R. H., Hampson, M., Krysatal, J. H., & Esterlis, I. (2018). Cerebellar and prefrontal cortical alterations in PTSD: Structural and functional evidence. *Chronic Stress, 2.*

Kardiner, A. (1941). The traumatic neuroses of war. *Psychosomatic Medicine. Monographs, 1*, Nos. 2 & 3.

Keane, T. M., Kolb, L. C., Kaloupek, D. G., Orr, S. P., Blanchard, E. B., Thomas, R. G., Hsieh, F. Y., & Lavori, P. W. (1998). Utility of psychophysiological measurement in the diagnosis of posttraumatic stress disorder: Results from a department of veterans affairs cooperative study. *Journal of Consulting and Clinical Psychology, 66*, 914–923.

Lanius, R. A., Brand, B., Vermetten, E., Frewen, P. A., & Spiegel, D. (2012). The dissociative subtype of posttraumatic stress disorder: Rationale, clinical and neurobiological evidence, and implications. *Depression and Anxiety, 29*, 701–708.

Lanius, R. A., Williamson, P. C., Boksman, K., Densmore, M., Gupta, M., Neufeld, R. W. J., Gati, J. S., & Menon, R. S. (2002). Brain activation during script-driven imagery induced dissociative responses in PTSD: A functional MRI investigation. *Biological Psychiatry, 52*, 305–311.

Lanius, R. A., Wolf, E. J., Miller, M. W., Frewen, P. A., Vermetten, E., Brand, B., & Spiegel, D. (2014). Chapter 13: The dissociative subtype of PTSD. In M. J. Friedman, T. M. Keane & P. A. Resick (Eds.), *The handbook of PTSD: Science and practice* (2nd ed., pp. 234–250). New York: The Guilford Press.

Leen-Feldner, E. W., Feldner, M. T., Knapp, A., Bunaciu, L., Blumenthal, H., & Amstadter, A. B. (2013). Offspring psychological and biological correlates of parental posttraumatic stress: Review of the literature and research agenda. *Clinical Psychology Review, 33*, 1106–1133.

Logue, M. W., van Rooij, S. J. H., Dennis, E. L., Davis, S. L., Hayes, J. P., Stevens, J. S., …, Moray, R. A. (2017). Smaller hippocampal volume in posttraumatic stress disorder: A multisite ENIGMA-PGC study: Subcortical volumetry results from posttraumatic stress disorder consortia. *Biological Psychiatry, 83*, 244–253.

Meakins, J. C., & Wilson, R. M. (1918). The effect of certain sensory stimulation on the respiratory rate in case of so-called "irritable heart". *Heart, 7*, 17–22.

Menon, V. (2011). Large-scale brain networks and psychopathology: A unifying triple network model. *Trends in Cognitive Sciences, 15*, 483–506.

Morris, M. C., Compas, B. E., & Garber, J. (2012). Relations among posttraumatic stress disorder, comorbid major depression, and HPA function: A systematic review and meta-analysis. *Clinical Psychology Review, 32*, 301–315.

Olff, M., & van Zuiden, M. (2017). Neuroendocrine and neuroimmune markers in PTSD: Pre-, peri- and post-trauma glucocorticoid and inflammatory dysregulation. *Current Opinion in Psychology, 14*, 132–137.

Orr, S. P., Lasko, N. B., Metzger, L. J., Berry, N. J., Ahern, C. E., & Pitman, R. K. (1998). Psychophysiologic assessment of women with posttraumatic stress disorder resulting from childhood sexual abuse. *Journal of Consulting and Clinical Psychology, 66*, 906–913.

Orr, S. P., Metzger, L. J., Miller, M. W., & Kaloupek, D. G. (2004). Psychophysiological assessment of PTSD. In J. P. Wilson & T. M. Keane (Eds.), *Assessing psychological trauma and PTSD: A handbook for practitioners* (2nd ed., pp. 289–343). New York: Guilford Press.

Philippi, C. L., Pessin, S., Reyna, L., Floyd, T., & Bruce, S. E. (2020). Cortical midline structures associated with rumination in women with PTSD. *Journal of Psychiatric Research, 131*, 69–76.

Pitman, R. K., Orr, S. P., Forgue, D. F., Altman, B., & deJong, J. (1990). Psychophysiologic responses to combat imagery of Vietnam veterans with posttraumatic stress disorder versus other anxiety disorders. *Journal of Abnormal Psychology, 99*, 49–54.

Pitman, R. K., Orr, S. P., Forgue, D. F., de Jong, J. B., & Claiborn, J. M. (1987). Psychophysiologic assessment of posttraumatic stress disorder imagery in Vietnam combat veterans. *Archives of General Psychiatry, 44*, 970–975.

Pitman, R. K., Rasmusson, A. M., Koenen, K. C., Shin, L., Orr, S. P., Gilbertson, M. W., Milad, M. R., & Liberzon, I. (2012). Biological studies of post-traumatic stress disorder. *Nature Reviews, 13*, 769–787.

Ramage, A. E., Litz, B., Resick, P. A., Woolsey, M. D., Dondanville, K. A., Young-McCaughan, S., Borah, A. M., Borah, E. V., Peterson, A. L., & Fox, P. T., and the STRONG STAR Consortium. (2016). Neurophysiology associated with danger-based and non-danger-based traumas in posttraumatic stress disorder. *Social Cognitive and Affective Neuroscience, 11*, 234–242.

Rasmusson, A. M., Kim, B. K., Lago, T. R., Brown, K., Ridgewell, C., & Shalev, A. Y. (2021). Chapter 10: Neurochemistry, neuroendocrinology, and neuroimmunology of PTSD. In M. J. Friedman, P. P. Schnurr & T. M. Keane (Eds.), *Handbook of PTSD: Science and practice* (3rd ed., pp. 168–191). New York: Guilford Press.

Sheerin, C. M., Lind, M. J., Bountress, K. E., Nugent, N. R., & Amstadter, A. B. (2017). The genetics and epigenetics of PTSD: Overview, recent advances, and future directions. *Current Opinion in Psychology, 14*, 5–11.

Stein, D. J., Koenen, K. C., Friedman, M. J., Hill, E., McLaughlin, K. A., Petukhova, M. et al. (2013). Dissociation in posttraumatic stress disorder: Evidence from the World Mental Health Surveys. *Biological Psychiatry, 73*, 302–312.

Steuwe, C., Lanius, R. A., & Frewen, P. A. (2012). Evidence for a dissociative subtype of PTSD by latent profile and confirmatory factor analyses in a civilian sample. *Depression and Anxiety, 29*, 689–700.

True, W. R., Rice, J., Eisen, S. A., Heath, A. C., Goldberg, J., Lyons, M. J., & Nowak, J. (1993). A twin study of genetic and environmental contributions to liability for posttraumatic stress symptoms. *Archives of General Psychiatry, 50*, 257–264.

Voisey, J., Young, R. M., Lawford, B. R., & Morris, C. P. (2014). Progress towards understanding the genetics of posttraumatic stress disorder. *Journal of Anxiety Disorders, 28*, 873–883.

Wolf, E. J., Lunney, C. A., Miller, M. W., Resick, P. A., Friedman, M. J., & Schnurr, P. P. (2012a). The dissociative subtype of PTSD: A replication and extension. *Depression and Anxiety, 29*, 679–688.

Wolf, E. J., Miller, M. W., Reardon, A. F., Ryabchenko, K. A., Castillo, D., & Freund, R. (2012b). A latent class analysis of dissociation and PTSD: Evidence for a dissociative subtype. *Archives of General Psychiatry, 69*, 698–705.

Yehuda, R., Lowy, M. T., Southwick, S. M., Shaffer, S., & Oiller, E. L. (1991). Increased number of gluco-corticoid receptor number in post-traumatic stress disorder. *American Journal of Psychiatry, 149*, 499–504.

5

Risk Factors for PTSD

Because people show varying responses to similar traumatic events, it is likely that the trauma itself is not solely responsible for causing posttrauma symptoms. This has led to a search for factors that may affect trauma response and recovery. Chapter 4 considered how trauma affects biological responses and, further, how biological responses might affect recovery from trauma. This chapter will cover how trauma responses are affected by personal or interpersonal variables prior to, during, or after the traumatic events being studied. Some of the variables may be considered basic demographics (fixed variables) such as the trauma survivors' race, age at the time of the trauma, or educational level. Some factors that influence recovery are individual factors such as trauma survivors' psychological history or prior experiences with trauma. The severity of the stressor and other factors occurring within the trauma may affect reactions and recovery. The way in which people respond cognitively and emotionally during the trauma may also affect how they react and recover. Finally, following the potentially traumatic event, there are variables that may affect how someone recovers or maintains their initial posttraumatic stress disorder (PTSD) symptoms.

For many decades, predictor studies were conducted after a traumatic event, sometimes years later, which could affect the participants' memories of their pretrauma functioning. This is especially important when measuring more subjective factors such as pretrauma distress, childhood environment, or life stressors, but somewhat less so for factual information such as age, gender, education, or ethnicity, although people may not remember facts like age at which the events occurred accurately either. More recently, studies have been conducted that assess participants both before and after traumatic events that can more clearly delineate the predictive

DOI: 10.4324/9780429317934-5

power of pretrauma variables, factors that occurred during the event (peritraumatic factors), or factors that occur after the traumatic event that might affect recovery and PTSD severity. Some variables like social support can change over time along with symptoms, so prospective studies are important to understand the relationship between these factors and outcomes. Much of the research on psychosocial risk factors has been contradictory, indicating there are no definitive risk factors that are always associated with PTSD. In fact, there could be combinations of risk factors that would be more reliable predictors, but the number of possible combinations is endless and could depend on the population being studied (Vogt et al., 2014). The rest of this chapter will focus on particularly large studies, meta-analyses that examine multiple studies, and longitudinal studies, with special notice of prospective studies assessing pre-traumatic factors.

Demographic Factors

Gender

Findings with regard to gender have been fairly consistent. Overall, women have a higher lifetime prevalence of PTSD than men (Breslau et al., 1991; Kessler et al., 1995; Weaver & Clum, 1995). In their national prevalence study of PTSD, Kessler et al. found that although women had higher rates of lifetime PTSD than men did, the results might be accounted for somewhat by the differences in their traumas. Although men were more likely than women to have experienced at least one trauma, women were more likely to have experienced as their worst event, an event likely to cause PTSD (e.g., rape).

In studying gender differences in PTSD, Breslau et al. (1997) found that there was a twofold difference in PTSD between women and men primarily due to age and trauma differences. They found an interaction such that women were more likely to experience PTSD if their trauma exposure occurred in childhood before the age of 15. They also found that young girls were more likely to have as their traumas rape, assault, or ongoing physical or sexual abuse, while boys were more likely to have experienced serious accidents or injury. Accidents and injuries were not as likely to lead to PTSD in trauma survivors of either gender while childhood sexual and physical abuse resulted in PTSD in 63% of the participants. Therefore, they concluded that younger age at the time of the trauma and the experience of interpersonal violence may contribute to the gender differences that have been observed. However, Breslau (2009) conducted a review of epidemiological studies and reported that while women are more likely to experience PTSD following traumatic events, the available studies indicate that the sex difference is not due to higher occurrence of sexual assault among women, prior traumatic experiences, preexisting depression or anxiety, or sex-related bias in reporting.

Lehavot et al. (2019) examined whether trauma type, stressful life events, and social support explain why women veterans have particularly high prevalence of PTSD compared to male veterans or female civilians. They examined a cross-sectional study of a very large sample regarding past-year PTSD as part of a National Epidemiologic Survey on Alcohol and Related Conditions. The authors conducted face-to-face interviews with 379 women veterans, over 20,000 women civilians, and 2,740 male veterans concerning history of trauma type (child abuse, interpersonal violence, combat), number of types of trauma, past-year stressful events, current social support, and current PTSD. Women veterans had higher rates of PTSD than female civilians or male veterans. Compared to the civilian women, female veterans were more likely to be older, White, with higher income, but also more likely to have been exposed to more types of trauma, interpersonal trauma, and past-year life stress. Compared to male veterans, female veterans were younger, were more likely to be White, reported child abuse and interpersonal violence, and were less likely to be married. There were no differences among the three groups in perceived social support. The differences were eliminated between the female groups by adjusting for differences in the number of trauma types; however, male and female veterans' differences in PTSD rates were reduced somewhat by adjusting for child abuse, interpersonal violence, and stressful life events but still remained significant. These studies indicate a gender difference in PTSD, but the explanations are contradictory and may depend on interactions between age and type of trauma.

There are two exceptions to the usual gender difference finding. One was in a study by Carlson et al. (2016) in which they studied an almost equal number of male and female patients and their family members ($n = 129$) who were hospitalized for severe trauma and then again two months later. They found no gender differences in their study of pretrauma, peritraumatic, or posttraumatic variables. Jacobson et al. (2015) examined a large sample of veterans (4,684 total) who were matched for gender as well as a large number of other variables including sexual assault history. They found that 6.7% of women and 6.1% of men had PTSD at the follow-up and that women did not have a different risk for developing PTSD than men after experiencing combat.

Age

Age effects are more difficult to determine because many studies include either children or adults but not the full age range. Many studies look back, and adult participants report on childhood trauma or family environment, which can be less accurate over time.

Schnurr et al. (2004) found that among Vietnam veterans, higher age at Vietnam entry was associated with lower risk of PTSD. The age of the person being studied appears to be associated with the level of trauma symptoms. Keane et al. (1998) also examined Vietnam veterans who were receiving psychological services and found that age on arrival in Vietnam also made a difference. Men with current PTSD were more likely to be younger at the time they went to Vietnam than men who never developed PTSD. Fontana and Rosenheck (1994) examined the veterans of three different wars: World War II, Korea, and Vietnam. They found that the older veterans were less symptomatic than the younger men, even after controlling for the effects of education, medical conditions, traumatic exposure, and in which war they served.

Age was the strongest risk factor for predicting global distress following trauma in a sample of 1,000 adults who were surveyed in four cities in the southern United States (Norris, 1992). Ten lifetime traumatic stressors were assessed. The young group included those 18–39. The middle group was 40–59, and the older group was 60+. The oldest group reported the least impact with regard to general stress and PTSD. Weaver and Clum (1995) conducted a meta-analysis, a statistical analysis of 50 studies on interpersonal violence. They found that age was not related to the impact of the trauma. However, across all of these studies, the mean age was 24, and the range was age 6–41. Therefore, the participants in these studies would have fallen in Norris's youngest group. Other epidemiology studies of adults have found that the oldest age groups have the lowest probability of PTSD (Kessler et al., 2005; Reynolds et al., 2016).

A number of researchers have conducted studies at set points in time following particular disasters, which circumvent the problem of varying lengths of time since exposure (Bolin & Klenow, 1982–1983; Huerta & Horton, 1978; Melick & Logue, 1985, 1986). All of these studies found that younger victims reported more family problems, emotional stress, and physical stress.

When age was not used as a linear variable, but groups were divided into younger, middle-aged, and elderly, some studies have found that the middle-aged (36–50) group were at the greatest risk for symptoms (Phifer, 1990; Price, 1978; Shore et al., 1986; Thompson et al., 1993). For example, in examining the effects of Hurricane Hugo, Thompson et al. (1993) found that experience with prior trauma, injuries, life threat, and personal loss did not vary by age, but the middle-aged people were most seriously affected with a range of outcomes (depression, anxiety, somatization, general stress, and traumatic stress). After examining several possible explanations, Thompson et al. proposed that the middle-aged groups have more burden placed upon them and hence more stress. They have greater responsibilities for both children and aging parents as well as greater societal and financial responsibilities. Community disasters increase the stress disproportionately in this age group.

Race/Ethnicity

Most studies have found that race is not associated with psychological impact of trauma (e.g., Breslau et al., 1997; Kessler et al., 1995). In the meta-analytic analysis of 50 studies of interpersonal violence, Weaver and Clum (1995) found that race was not associated with reactions following interpersonal trauma. However, there have been some exceptions. In a study of a range of traumas, Norris (1992) found that overall, there was higher stress and posttraumatic stress among White subjects. However, there was also an interaction of race and gender such that the strongest psychological reactions were found among African-American men. In the National Vietnam Veterans Readjustment Study (Kulka et al., 1990), it was found that Hispanic individuals had the highest rate of current PTSD (28%) followed by African-Americans (21%) and then Whites/others (14%). Schnurr et al. (2004) studied risk factors from the National Vietnam Veterans Readjustment Study and the Hawaiian Vietnam Veterans Project including comparing veterans who never had PTSD with those with lifetime PTSD. They found that being Hispanic rather than White was associated with higher risk of PTSD, while being Native Hawaiian or Japanese American was associated with lower risk of PTSD.

Davis et al. (2012) examined Black vs. White military veteran survivors of Hurricane Katrina. There were many other variables that covaried with race and that were also predictors, such as employment status, number of prior lifetime traumatic experiences, number of Katrina-related traumatic stressors, and current social support. When they controlled for all of the covariates, there was still a race difference in new-onset PTSD, but only for veterans with combat experience. As with this study, most studies have interactions between risk factors, and the most compelling studies have examined participants before and after exposure to trauma.

Trauma Type and Trauma History

Although type of trauma or prior history of trauma is not a fixed variable, it is also not something that can easily be studied prospectively. Studies indicate that military trauma is more likely to result in PTSD than civilian trauma, although that could be confounded with gender, education, and age. Sexual assault and particularly child sexual abuse appear to be risk factors for further trauma and PTSD. Gidycz et al. (1993) conducted a prospective study with college women and found that those with a history of abuse were 1.5–2 times more likely to be victimized during their initial academic quarter of participation in their longitudinal study than women without a history of abuse.

Ruch et al. (1980) examined the presence of 11 life stressors during the year prior to a rape and found a curvilinear relationship. Women who had experienced major life changes were most traumatized, women with no changes were intermediate, and those with minor changes were the least traumatized. Apparently, experience with some life stress may have an inoculating effect, but too great a level of stress interferes with the development of coping methods needed to deal with an event as traumatic as rape.

Resnick et al. (1993) conducted a national prevalence study of over 4,000 adult women and found that the rate of PTSD (past six months) was significantly higher among crime versus noncrime traumas (26% versus 9%). History of traumas that included direct threat to life or receipt of injury were risk factors for PTSD.

Ruch and Leon (1983) evaluated rape victims within 48 hours post-crime and then again at two weeks post-crime. They found that women with no history of prior victimization showed a decrease in their trauma scores, while those with prior victimization exhibited an increase in trauma scores across the two weeks. They concluded that women who were multiple-incident victims were especially at risk for delayed responses.

Several studies on rape have examined the effect of prior victimization of any type, not just prior rapes. Burgess and Holmstrom (1978) conducted a four-to-six-year follow-up of 81 women originally seen at a hospital emergency room. They reported differences in recovery depending upon their history of victimization: 47% of participants with no prior history of victimization recovered within months and only 14% were not yet recovered, while only 53% of victims with such a history felt recovered upon follow-up. Both economic stress and other chronic stressors also impacted recovery. Functional and emotional social support also made an impact. With social support, 45% reported they recovered in months, but without it, none reported recovering in months. At the long-term follow-up, 20% with social support were not recovered, while 53% without social report had still not recovered.

Garfin et al. (2020) studied the effects of prior stress and trauma in childhood and adulthood after the Boston Marathon bombings. Both childhood and adult traumas were associated with greater post-bombing acute stress, and in a second wave of data collection, childhood, adulthood, and recent (past six months) traumas were associated with post-bombing PTSD symptoms.

Meta-analyses and Systematic Reviews

Brewin et al. (2000) conducted a meta-analysis of 77 studies. Risk factors were included if they were assessed in at least four of the studies, resulting in 14 risk factor variables (gender, younger age, low socioeconomic status, lower education, lower intelligence, minority race, psychiatric history, childhood abuse, other prior trauma, other adverse childhood events, family psychiatric history, trauma severity, lack of social support, and life stress). While all of the predictors were significant, none of the pretrauma variables were strong predictors of PTSD. Trauma severity, life stress, and lack of social support had larger effects than any of the pretrauma variables. There were some interactions between variables, however. For example, with regard to gender, the researchers found that in studies including both genders, military samples did not show gender to be a risk factor for PTSD, while civilian samples did. In fact, military versus civilian samples proved to be the biggest predictor of PTSD.

In military samples, lack of education, younger age at the time of the trauma, minority race, trauma severity, and lack of social support were more important than in civilian samples.

Ozer et al. (2003) conducted a meta-analysis after reviewing thousands of studies as a follow-up to the Brewin et al. (2000) study. While there was overlap in the studies, Ozer et al. included 21 studies not included in the Brewin et al. study, and two predictors not included before were peritraumatic emotions and peritraumatic dissociation. There were 68 studies that met the criteria for including seven predictors: prior trauma, prior psychological adjustment, family history of psychopathology, posttrauma social support, perceived threat during the trauma, peritraumatic emotional responses, and peritraumatic dissociation. Again, all variables were significantly related to PTSD symptoms but with small effects. The strongest of the group of variables was peritraumatic dissociation, which was still a small effect. In a study of 469 firefighters in Australia, McFarlane (1989) found that a past history of treatment of psychological disorders was a better predictor of posttrauma symptoms than the degree of exposure to the disaster or the losses sustained. Prior psychiatric symptoms were also found to predict PTSD among Vietnam veterans (Kulka et al., 1990).

Digangi et al. (2013) conducted a systematic review of 54 prospective and longitudinal studies, focusing on six categories of preexisting factors that predicted later PTSD: (1) cognitive abilities, (2) coping and response styles, (3) personality factors, (4) psychopathology, (5) psychophysiological factors, and (6) social ecological factors. The participants included police officers, military members, veterans, firefighters, children, pregnant women, and undergraduates who were first assessed pretrauma. First, with regard to cognitive abilities, a range of measures were used from intelligence quotient (four studies) to other forms of cognitive functioning such as retrieval of autobiographical memories, negative appraisals of self, cognitive abilities with regard to military trainability, extinction learning, and processing speed and memory. In all cases, lower cognitive ability, no matter how it was measured at pretrauma, was associated with increased PTSD symptoms at posttrauma.

Prospective Studies

Demographic Variables

Several studies have focused on intelligence or education prospectively. Breslau et al. (2006) conducted a study of intelligence, anxiety, and conduct problems with 713 children at age 6 and then again at age 17 for both exposure to trauma and PTSD. They found that children with higher ratings of externalizing problems were at increased risk for trauma exposure and later PTSD. Children with anxiety disorders were more likely to have PTSD at 17. Children with an IQ greater than 115 at age 6 were at decreased risk for both traumatic events and PTSD. Kremen et al. (2007) examined Vietnam era twins and cognitive ability scores. The study examined the Armed Forces Qualification Test of cognitive ability that was administered just before military induction (mean age 20) and PTSD years later (mean age 42) among over 2,000 veterans who were exposed to potentially traumatic events. They found that the highest cognitive ability quartile had a significantly lower risk of PTSD than the lowest ability quartile. They concluded that preexposure cognitive ability served as either a risk or protective factor for PTSD.

Shalev et al. (2019) reported on 2,473 civilian trauma survivors admitted to ten acute care centers in six countries as part of the International Consortium to Predict PTSD. Participants were assessed within 60 days of trauma exposure and again 4–15 months later. The purpose of the study was to examine the likelihood of PTSD at follow-up given early predictors. At the follow-up, 9% of men and 16% of women met the criteria for PTSD. Early PTSD symptom severity was a strong predictor of later PTSD, but adding female gender, lower education, and prior exposure to interpersonal trauma increased the prediction of PTSD. Weaver and Clum (1995) in a meta-analysis of 50 studies did not find that either socioeconomic status or education were related to distress. Overall, it appears that if there are socioeconomic or educational differences, they may be indirect such that those with lower income and education may be exposed to more traumatic stressors.

Pretrauma Psychological History

US service members participated in the Millennium Cohort Study from 2001 to 2003 with follow-ups up to 2008 and a deployment occurring between the first baseline and the follow-up (Sandweiss et al., 2011). In this prospective study of over 22,000 eligible participants, 1,840 (8.1%) screened positive for PTSD and 1% sustained a physical injury during deployment. The odds of screening positive for PTSD were more than twice as likely for those with a history of predeployment psychiatric distress (including psychiatric history, use of psychotropic medications, and stressful life events) compared to those who were injured during deployment although both were associated with later PTSD. The other variables that were associated with post-deployment PTSD included female gender, racial minority status, lower educational level, and deployment related variables (e.g., combat exposure, length of deployment).

While several studies in this chapter have looked at pretrauma psychiatric problems, two studies examined anger in particular to see if it is cause or effect–or both. Anger is an important target for study because it is linked to decreases in social and occupational functioning and associated with risk for poor cardiac functioning. Anger is also associated with increases in interpersonal violence. Meffert et al. (2008) conducted a prospective study of 180 police academy trainees. Only combat veterans and prior first responders were excluded. They were assessed again 12 months after beginning active police duty. At baseline, none of the participants had PTSD or other psychological disorders. Social support at baseline was associated with social support at 12 months. Trait anger assessed during academy training was associated with state anger at 12 months, and state anger at 12 months was highly related to PTSD symptoms (after removing anger items from the measure) after controlling for trait anger at baseline and other variables. The conclusion was that trait anger is a risk factor for PTSD symptoms and that PTSD symptoms are also related to an increase in state anger.

A second study, conducted in the Netherlands, also examined anger prospectively (Lommen et al., 2014). In that study, 249 Dutch soldiers were tested two months before and two and nine months after deployment to Afghanistan. Trait anger, neuroticism, and PTSD symptom severity were assessed at all three assessments along with deployment stressors. On average, the soldiers reported 14 warzone related stressors. They found that trait anger before deployment predicted PTSD symptom severity two months after deployment and indirectly at nine months. However, trait anger at two months post-deployment did not predict PTSD severity at nine months, nor did PTSD at two months predict trait anger at nine months. Perhaps the differences between the two studies is that this second study continued to measure trait anger instead of switching to state anger in response to their experiences.

Constans et al. (2012) took a somewhat different approach to exploring preexisting psychological problems as a predictor. They examined Department of Veterans Affairs medical records and found that those with a mental health diagnosis prior to Hurricane Katrina were likely to have more severe PTSD over two years later. They also studied negative cognitions following the hurricane. They found that those with negative cognitions post-Katrina were strongly associated with higher PTSD severity and were also associated with pre-hurricane mental illness, even after removing the effects of level of stress exposure, social support, and damage to property. In a second study, Sullivan et al. (2013) studied 249 veterans with and 250 veterans without preexisting mental illness after Katrina. They adjusted for demographics and exposure-related stressors and found the odds of screening positive for any new mental disorder (PTSD, depression, generalized anxiety disorder, or panic disorder) were 6.8 times greater for those with preexisting mental illness compared with those without preexisting mental illness. Among those with preexisting PTSD, the odds of screening positive for any new mental illness were 11.9 times greater; among those with schizophrenia, 9.1 times greater; and among those with affective disorders, 4.4 times greater.

Coping and Cognitions

In a large meta-analysis of 54 prospective and longitudinal studies (DiGangi et al., 2013), eight studies examined coping and response styles pretrauma such as rumination, emotion-focused avoidance, and cognitive coping. All were preexisting risk factors for PTSD symptoms at the posttrauma period. Personality and other symptom factors, examined in 14 studies, also included a wide range of preexisting variables including negative emotions or appraisals, neuroticism, hostility, anxiety, self-esteem, and dissociation. The only variable that did not show a relationship with later PTSD symptoms was self-esteem. Prior psychopathology was a bit more complicated because the majority of the 54 studies included in the review did not examine prior psychological disorders, including prior PTSD. Therefore, it is difficult to tell if having a disorder prior to a subsequent trauma is actually a risk factor or the result of prior experiences. Nevertheless, 19 of 23 studies that used psychopathology as a risk factor found it to have an effect on subsequent PTSD symptoms.

Su and Chen (2018) studied pretrauma cognitions among university students in Taiwan to see how they might affect trauma responses. They initially assessed 821 students with scales they developed that were assumed to be trauma-related cognitions (e.g. "The world is completely dangerous" or "I am totally incompetent") or depressive cognitions from an established scale. Two months later, 592 completed a second assessment and, of those, 97 had experienced a traumatic event; most commonly an earthquake (29%), loved one experiencing a life-threatening event (20%), sudden death of a close friend or loved one (18%), transportation accident (13%), and a number of other less common events. After controlling for preexisting variables such as gender, prior trauma, and history of depression or anxiety, they examined whether trauma or depressive cognitions were risk factors for acute stress disorder symptoms (immediate PTSD symptoms). They found that preexisting PTSD-related cognitions, but not depressive cognitions, predicted PTSD symptoms at the follow-up time point.

Social ecological factors refer to variables outside of the person themselves (DiGangi et al., 2013). In the meta-analysis, these variables included family of origin, stressors outside of the family like work or finances, and social support beyond the family. The majority of the studies found that preexisting problems with social support within or outside of the family were risk factors for PTSD. An important conclusion from the review of the literature is that variables that were previously thought of as outcomes of traumatic events are likely to be preexisting variables related to subsequent PTSD. However, these preexisting variables may themselves have been subsequent to even earlier traumas as indicated by some of the other studies that examined prior trauma history.

Peritraumatic Factors

Threat and Exposure

A number of studies have included peritraumatic (occurring during the trauma) factors including injury, level of threat, or peritraumatic dissociation. Vogt et al. (2011) studied predeployment, deployment, and postdeployment risk factors among 579 veterans of the wars in Iraq and Afghanistan to determine direct and indirect risk factors as pathways to PTSD symptoms. Models were calculated for women and men separately. They found that the majority of risk pathways were similar for women and men. For women, perceived threat during deployment, postdeployment stressors, and postdeployment social support all had direct effects on PTSD symptoms, although predeployment stressors did not. However, prior stressors had an indirect effect through postdeployment stressors, and warfare exposure had an indirect effect on PTSD through perceived threat. For men, prior stressors again did not have a direct effect on PTSD symptoms, but perceived threat, postdeployment stressors, and postdeployment social support all had direct effects on PTSD symptoms. For both men and women, predeployment stressors affected the relationship between warfare exposure and relationship concerns, and between warfare exposure and PTSD symptoms.

Yuan et al. (2011) studied protective, rather than risk factors, and found similar variables to be important but in the inverse direction. They studied 233 police officers during training and then again two years later. White race, lower critical incident exposure during police service, better social support, greater assumptions of benevolence of the world, and better social adjustment during training remained predictive of lower PTSD symptoms after two years of police service.

In another study of 774 US Army soldiers who were assessed prior to and after deployment, Franz et al. (2013) examined soldiers' previous life stressors, deployment history, current (predeployment) PTSD symptoms, deployment preparedness, and unit cohesion. Structural equation modeling revealed that predeployment PTSD symptom severity, prior warzone deployment, unit cohesion, and preparedness were each independently associated with deployment threat appraisal, even after taking into account combat intensity. Deployment threat appraisal was associated with postdeployment PTSD severity. In other words, the predeployment variables had an indirect effect on postdeployment PTSD but did affect threat appraisal during deployment.

By coincidence, 180 students at the University of Haifa were participating in research two weeks before a suicide bomb explosion on a bus enroute to the university. These students agreed to participate in research on their reactions (Gil & Caspi, 2006). One week after the attack the students were asked about their proximity to the explosion and their perceived threat. One month after the attack they completed the same measures they had before the attack on personality traits and coping style. At six months postexplosion they were assessed for PTSD. The students were divided into two groups based on their PTSD status; 31 (17%) met full criteria for PTSD while 149 (83%) did not. The two groups did not differ on age, gender, marital status, or country of origin. Proximity to the attack and perceived threat were associated with PTSD. When all of the variables were examined in a model, increased risk of PTSD was predicted by direct exposure and indirect exposure to the bomb as well as preattack harm avoidance personality style. Perceived threat was not associated with actual exposure and was not predictive of PTSD.

Effects of Injury

As mentioned earlier, extent of injury during the trauma was a significant predictor in Sandweiss et al. (2011). The level of exposure during the World Trade Center collapse (Pietrzak et al., 2014) and level of peritraumatic dissociation (Ozer et al., 2003) were also predictors of later PTSD. Hodgins et al. (2001) conducted a prospective study of junior police officers and found that severity of incident exposure and peritraumatic dissociation were both predictive of posttraumatic stress symptoms. On the other hand, as reviewed earlier, in a study of firefighters in Australia, McFarlane (1989) found that a past history of treatment of psychological disorders was a better predictor of posttrauma symptoms than the degree of exposure to the disaster or the losses sustained.

In order to clarify the relationships between objective and subjective measures of injury severity and later PTSD, Gabert-Quillen et al. (2011) recruited 65 trauma victims who had been hospitalized for traumatic injuries to participate in a longitudinal study and were able to assess 45 through a three-month follow-up. Objective injury severity was coded from medical charts and a phone interview that also included subjective injury, peritraumatic dissociation, and peritraumatic distress. At six weeks and three months posttrauma, participants were mailed packets of questionnaires including injury recovery and posttrauma reactions. They found that non-White and younger participants reported higher PTSD symptoms. These two variables were covaried in the remainder of analyses. They found that objective and subjective reports of injury were not related and that objective injury severity was not related to PTSD symptoms at six weeks and three months. Subjective injury severity was consistently and positively predictive of PTSD at both time points. They also found interesting interactions. Being severely injured and being a medium-high dissociator was related to more PTSD symptoms while being severely injured but a low dissociator was associated with fewer PTSD symptoms.

Posttrauma Factors

Research on posttrauma factors, especially in cross-sectional studies, has often focused on social support, but it appears that pretrauma social support is predictive of posttrauma support and lack of social support before traumatic events may start a resource loss spiral that is associated with problems in recovery. Conservation of resources (COR) theory (Hobfoll, 2001) has been used to explain how changes in resources can explain adjustment following trauma. Using that model, Littleton et al. (2009) prospectively studied 293 female students who were enrolled at Virginia Tech at the time of a mass shooting. They had already completed an assessment for a different study on sexual assault at the time of the shooting and were recontacted to be assessed at two and six months postshooting. They hypothesized that those with fewer interpersonal resources (poorer social support) prior to the shooting and more psychological distress would experience more loss of resources. Aside from measuring psychological symptoms at pretrauma, they also received a measure of perceived social support. After the shooting they were assessed for level of exposure and relationship with those who were wounded or killed, PTSD symptoms, and a measure of resource loss (life direction, optimism, interpersonal resources, etc). In keeping with the COR model, loss of valued interpersonal or intrapersonal resources predicted PTSD symptoms later. And with two to six month resource loss, it demonstrated a loss spiral with greater PTSD symptoms. Preshooting distress and less social support predicted resource loss postshooting.

In the Carlson et al. (2016) study that was mentioned at the beginning of the chapter, severely injured hospitalized patients were assessed 1–14 days posttrauma exposure and two months later. Their analysis assessed the predictive role of the variables in the order of pretrauma, trauma severity, acute stress symptoms, and posttrauma life stress and social support. After accounting for the pretrauma variables, including prior history of trauma, the risk factors with the strongest relationship to posttraumatic symptoms were acute stress symptoms, posttrauma life stress, and posttrauma social support.

Maguen et al. (2009) were interested in studying the effects of work environment on PTSD outcomes among police over their first year. Participants were assessed first during training at the police academy and then 12 months after police training. The model they examined included gender, ethnicity, traumatic exposure prior to entering the academy, current negative life events, critical incident exposure (number of times exposed) over the last year, and routine work environment stress (a total score summarizing management and administration, supervisors, equipment, training, boredom, role conflict, peers, work-related discrimination, shift work, and public attitudes). Several variables had a direct effect on PTSD symptoms: ethnicity, negative life events in past 12 months, critical incident exposure, and work environment. Work environment was most strongly associated with PTSD symptoms. They also found that routine work environment stress mediated the relationship between critical incident exposure and PTSD symptoms and between current negative life events and PTSD symptoms. Although the work environment could be construed as a form of social support, it is much broader and includes operational problems as well as interpersonal relationships.

Summary

Pretrauma and peritrauma variables appear to have varying effects on recovery from traumatic events. Among the demographic variables, gender is the most consistent predictor, although it tends to be confounded with type of trauma. Being older at the time of the trauma tends to be a predictor of better recovery, although middle-aged people with more responsibilities to children and parents may be a particularly stressed age group. Race/ethnicity varied quite a bit across studies and needs to be studied further. However, race and ethnicity also need to be disentangled from education, systemic support, and age at the time of the trauma. Prior psychiatric problems and emotions such as anger were predictors in several of the studies conducted prospectively.

Traumatic stress effects appear to be cumulative, especially in military and veteran samples as well as first responders. Childhood sexual abuse history tends to be a predictor of worse reactions to adult traumas, and adult traumas impact reactions and recovery to subsequent events. The type of trauma and level of exposure within the event is a consistent predictor of reactions and recovery, and assaultive injuries have been a predictor in several studies. Pre- and posttrauma cognitive reactions and peritraumatic dissociation appear to be strong predictors of severity of reactions. Poor social support is a risk factor both pre- and posttrauma exposure, and more research is needed to disentangle the relationship between them. More prospective research with different populations is needed to determine the causal nature of variables in order to screen people for potential support or intervention. At this point, with thousands of studies conducted, it can be concluded that there is no one predictor that is universal as a risk factor for PTSD. Many variables and combinations of variables may account for risk factors for PTSD in addition to biological vulnerability.

References

Bolin, R., & Klenow, D. (1982–1983). Response of elderly to disaster: An age stratified analysis. *International Journal of Aging and Human Development, 16*, 283–296.

Breslau, N. (2009). The epidemiology of trauma, PTSD, and other posttrauma disorders. *Trauma Violence Abuse, 10*, 198–210.

Breslau, N., Davis, G. C., Andreski, P., & Peterson, E. (1991). Traumatic events and posttraumatic stress disorder in an urban population of young adults. *Archives of General Psychiatry, 48*, 216–222.

Breslau, N., Davis, G., Andreski, P., Peterson, E., & Schultz, L. (1997). Sex differences in posttraumatic stress disorder. *Archives of General Psychiatry, 54*, 1044–1048.

Breslau, N., Lucia, V. C., & Alvarado, G. F. (2006). Intelligence and other predisposing factors in exposure to trauma and posttraumatic stress disorder. *Archives of General Psychiatry, 63*, 1238–1245.

Brewin, C. R., Andrews, B., & Valentine, J. D. (2000). Meta-analysis of risk factors for posttraumatic stress disorder in trauma-exposed adults. *Journal of Consulting and Clinical Psychology, 68*, 748–766.

Burgess, A. W., & Holmstrom, L. L. (1978). Recovery from rape and prior stress. *Research in Nursing and Health, 1*, 165–174.

Carlson, E. B., Palmieri, P. A., Field, N. P., Dalenberg, C. J., Macia, K. S., & Spain D. A. (2016). Contributions of risk and protective factors to prediction of psychological symptoms after traumatic experiences. *Comprehensive Psychiatry, 69*, 106–115.

Constans, J. I., Vasterling, J. J., Deitch, E., Han, X., Tharp, A. L. T., Davis, T. D., & Sullivan, G. (2012). Pre-Katrina mental illness, postdisaster negative cognitions, and PTSD symptoms in male veterans following Hurricane Katrina. *Psychological Trauma: Theory, Research, Practice, and Policy, 4*, 568–577.

Davis, T. D., Sullivan, G., Vasterling, J. J., Tharp, A. L. T., Han, X., Deitch, E. A., & Constans, J. I. (2012). Racial variations in postdisaster PTSD among veteran survivors of Hurricane Katrina. *Psychological Trauma: Theory, Research, Practice and Policy, 4*, 447–456.

DiGangi, J. A., Gomez, D., Mendoza, L., Jason, L. A., Keys, C. B., & Koenen, K. C. (2013). Pretrauma risk factors for posttraumatic stress disorder: A systematic review of the literature. *Clinical Psychology Review, 33*, 728–744.

Fontana, A., & Rosenheck, R. (1994). Traumatic war stressors and psychiatric symptoms among World War II, Korean, and Vietnam war veterans. *Psychology and Aging, 9*, 27–33.

Franz, M. R., Wolf, E. J., MacDonald, H. Z., Marx, B. P., Proctor, S. P., & Vasterling, J. J. (2013). Relationships among predeployment risk factors, warzone-threat appraisal, and postdeployment PTSD symptoms. *Journal of Traumatic Stress, 26*, 498–506.

Gabert-Quillen, C. A., Fallon, W., & Delahanty, D. L. (2011). PTSD after traumatic injury: An investigation of the impact of injury severity and peritraumatic moderators. *Journal of Health Psychology, 16*, 678–687.

Garfin, D. R., Holman, A., & Silver, R. C. (2020). Exposure to prior negative life events and responses to the Boston Marathon bombings. *Psychological Trauma: Theory, Research, Practice, and Policy, 12*, 320–329.

Gidycz, C. A., Coble, C. N., Latham, L., & Layman, M. J. (1993). A sexual assault experience in adulthood and prior victimization experiences: A prospective analysis. *Psychology of Women Quarterly, 17*, 151–168.

Gil, S., & Caspi, Y. (2006). Personality traits, coping style, and perceived threat as predictors of posttraumatic stress disorder after exposure to a terrorist attack: A prospective study. *Psychosomatic Medicine, 68*, 904–909.

Hobfoll, S. E. (2001). The influence of culture, community, and the nested-self in the stress process: Advancing conservation of resources theory. *Applied Psychology: An International Review, 50*, 337–421.

Hodgins, G. A., Creamer, M., & Bell, R. (2001). Risk factors for posttrauma reactions in police officer: A longitudinal study. *The Journal of Nervous and Mental Disease, 189*, 541–547.

Huerta, F., & Horton, R. (1978). Coping behavior of elderly flood victim. *Gerontologists, 18*, 541–546.

Jacobson, I., Donoho, C., Crum-Cianflone, N., & Maguen, S. (2015). Longitudinal assessment of gender differences in the development of PTSD among US military personnel deployed in support of the operations in Iraq and Afghanistan. *Journal of Psychiatric Research, 68*, 30–36.

Keane, T. M., Kolb, L. C., Kaloupek, D. G., Orr, S. P., Blanchard, E. B., Thomas, R. G., Hsieh, F. Y., & Lavori, P. W. (1998). Utility of psychophysiological measurement in the diagnosis of posttraumatic stress disorder: Results from a department of veterans affairs cooperative study. *Journal of Consulting and Clinical Psychology, 66*, 914–923.

Kessler, R., Berglund, P., Demler, O., Jin, R., Merikangas, K., & Walters, E. (2005). Lifetime prevalence and age-of-onset distributions of DSM-IV disorders in the National Comorbidity Survey Replication. *Archives of General Psychiatry, 62*, 593–602.

Kessler, R., Sonnega, A., Bromet, E., Hughes, M., & Nelson, C. (1995). Post-traumatic stress disorder in the National Comorbidity Survey. *Archives of General Psychiatry, 52*, 1048–1060.

Kremen, W. S., Koenen, K. C., Boake, C., Purcell, S., Eisen, S. A., Franz, C. E., Tsuang, M. T., & Lyons, M. J. (2007). Pretrauma cognitive ability and risk for posttraumatic stress disorder: A twin study. *Archives of General Psychiatry, 64*, 361–368.

Kulka, R. A., Schlenger, W. E., Fairbank, J. A., Hough, R. L., Jordan, B. K., Marmar, C. R., & Weiss, D. S. (1990). *Trauma and the Vietnam war generation.* New York: Brunner/Mazel.

Lehavot, K., Goldberg, S. B., Chen, J. A., Katon, J. G., Glass, J. E., Fortney, J. C., Simpson, T. L. & Schnurr, P. P. (2019). Do trauma type, stressful life events, and social support explain women.

Littleton, H., Grills-Taquechel, A., & Axsom, D. (2009). Resource loss as a predictor of posttrauma symptoms among college women following the mass shooting at Virginia Tech. *Violence and Victims, 24*, 669–686.

Lommen, M. J. J., Engelhard, I. M., van de Schoot, R., & van den Hout, M. A. (2014). Anger: Cause or consequence of posttraumatic stress? A prospective study of Dutch soldiers. *Journal of Traumatic Stress, 27*, 200–207.

Maguen, S., Metzler, T. J., McCaslin, S. E., Inslicht, S. S., Henn-Haase, C., Neylan, T. C., & Marmar, C. R. (2009). Routine work environment stress and PTSD symptoms in police officers. *Journal of Nervous and Mental Disease, 197*, 754–760.

McFarlane, A. C. (1989). The aetiology of post-traumatic morbidity: Predisposing, precipitating and perpetuating factors. *British Journal of Psychiatry, 154*, 221–228.

Meffert, S. M., Metzler, T. J., Henn-Haase, C., McCaslin, S., Inslicht, S., Chemtob, C., Neylan, T., & Marmar, C. R. (2008). A prospective study of trait anger and PTSD symptoms in police. *Journal of Traumatic Stress, 21*, 410–416.

Melick, M., & Logue, J. (1985, 1986). The effect of disaster on the health and well-being of older women. *International Journal of Aging and Human Development, 21*, 27–38.

Norris, F. H. (1992). Epidemiology of trauma: Frequency and impact of different potentially traumatic events on different demographic groups. *Journal of Consulting and Clinical Psychology, 60*, 409–418.

Ozer E. J., Best S. R., Lipsey T. L., & Weiss D. S. (2003). Predictors of posttraumatic stress disorder and symptoms in adults: A meta-analysis. *Psychological Bulletin, 129*, 52–73.

Phifer, J. (1990). Psychological distress and somatic symptoms after natural disaster: Differential vulnerability among older adults. *Psychology and Aging, 5*, 412–420.

Pietrzak, R. H., Feder, A., Singh, R., Schechter, C. B., Bromet, E. J., Katz, C. L., Reissman, D. B., Ozbay F., Sharma, V., Crane, M., Harrison, D., Herbert, R., Levin, S. M., Luft B. J., Moline, J. M., Stellman, J. M., Udasin, I. G., Landrigan, P. J., & Southwick, S. M., (2014). Trajectories of PTSD risk and resilience in World Trade Center responders: An 8-year prospective cohort study. *Psychological Medicine, 44*, 205–219.

Price, J. (1978). Some age-related effects of the 1974 Brisbane floods. *Australian and New Zealand Journal of Psychiatry, 12*, 55–58.

Resnick, H. S., Kilpatrick, D. G., Dansky, B. S., Saunders, B. E., & Best, C. L. (1993). Prevalence of civilian trauma and posttraumatic stress disorder in a representative national sample of women. *Journal of Consulting and Clinical Psychology, 61*, 984–991.

Reynolds, K., Pietrzak, R. H., Mackenzie, C. S., Chou, K. L., & Sareen, J. (2016). Posttraumatic stress disorder across the adult lifespan: Findings from a nationally representative survey. *American Journal of Geriatric Psychiatry, 24*, 81–93.

Ruch, L. O., Chandler, S. M., & Harter, R. A. (1980). Life change and rape impact. *Journal of Health and Social Behavior, 21*, 248–260.

Ruch, L. O., & Leon, J. J. (1983). Sexual assault trauma and trauma change. *Women and Health, 8*, 5–21.

Sandweiss, D. A., Slymen, D. J., LeardMann, C. A., Smith, B., White, M. R., Boyko, E. J., et al. (2011). Preinjury psychiatric status, injury severity, and postdeployment posttraumatic stress disorder. *Archives of General Psychiatry, 68*, 496–504.

Schnurr, P. P., Lunney, C. A., & Sengupta, A. (2004). Risk factors for the development versus maintenance of posttraumatic stress disorder. *Journal of Traumatic Stress, 17*, 85–95.

Shalev, A. Y., Gevonden, M., …, Koenen, K. C. (2019). Estimating the risk of PTSD in recent trauma survivors: Results of the International Consortium to Predict PTSD (ICPP). *World Psychiatry, 18*, 77–87.

Shore, J., Tatum, E., & Vollmer, W. (1986). Psychiatric reactions to disaster: The Mount St. Helen's experience. *American Journal of Psychiatry, 143*, 590–595.

Su, Y.-J., & Chen, S.-H. (2018). Negative cognitions prior to trauma predict acute posttraumatic stress disorder symptomatology. *Journal of Traumatic Stress, 31*, 14–24.

Sullivan, G., Vasterling, J. J., Han, X., Tetan Tharp, A., Davis, T., Deitch, E. A., & Constans, J. I. (2013). Preexisting mental illness and risk for developing a new disorder after Hurricane Katrina. *Journal of Nervous and Mental Disease, 201*, 161–166.

Thompson, M. P., Norris, F. H., & Hanecek, B. (1993). Age differences in the psychological consequences of Hurricane Hugo. *Psychology and Aging, 8*, 606–616.

Vogt, D. S., King, D. W., & King, L. A. (2014). Risk pathways for PTSD: Making sense of the literature. In M. J. Friedman, T. M. Keane & P. A. Resick (Eds.), *Handbook of PTSD* (2nd ed.) (pp. 146–165). New York: Guilford Press.

Vogt, D., Smith, B., Elwy, R., Martin, J., Schultz, M. Drainoni, M.-L., & Eisen, S. (2011). Predeployment, deployment, and postdeployment risk factors for posttraumatic stress symptomatology in female and male OEF/OIF veterans. *Journal of Abnormal Psychology, 120,* 819–831.

Weaver, T., & Clum, G. (1995). Psychological distress associated with interpersonal violence: A meta analysis. *Clinical Psychology Review, 15,* 115–140.

Yuan, C., Wang, Z., Inslicht, S. S., McCaslin, S. E., Metzler, T. J., Henn-Haase, C., Apfel, B. A., Tong, H., Neylan, T. C., Fang, Y., & Marmar, C. R. (2011). Protective factors for posttraumatic stress disorder symptoms in a prospective study of police officers. *Psychiatry Research, 188,* 45–50.

6

Treatment of PTSD and Other Trauma-Related Disorders

Appropriate treatment for trauma depends upon a number of factors. Many people who have experienced a traumatic event recover naturally and do not need psychological or psychiatric treatment at all. Having supportive family and friends may be sufficient. For those experiencing some reactions to the trauma but not meeting criteria for a specific disorder such as posttraumatic stress disorder (PTSD) or depression, general counseling or psychotherapy may be helpful. These types of therapy provide support, empathy, and an environment in which a person can explore the meaning of the event. For more severe and chronic reactions, more specific interventions may be necessary. Comorbidity of two or more disorders also may complicate the treatment picture. This chapter will describe approaches to treatment that are offered in response to trauma, with a focus on evidence-based treatments recommended in clinical practice guidelines. More attention will be given to cognitive behavioral therapies because these therapy procedures have been researched the most and have the most evidence supporting their use. Nearly all of the available research and specific treatments have focused on PTSD rather than other trauma-related disorders, although many studies have examined treatment outcomes for comorbid symptoms beyond those of PTSD. What is extremely promising is that individuals can and do recover from the effects of trauma, even after suffering for many years.

DOI: 10.4324/9780429317934-6

Clinical Practice Guidelines for the Treatment of PTSD

Several organizations release clinical practice guidelines to inform mental health providers about the current state of the evidence for psychological interventions and recommend best practices. We will first provide an overview of the treatments recommended for PTSD across clinical practice guidelines. Later we will describe some of the more strongly research-supported therapies in more detail.

Overall, guidelines from the American Psychological Association (APA, 2017), the International Society for Traumatic Stress Studies (ISTSS, 2018), the US Department of Veterans Affairs and Department of Defense (VA/DoD, 2023), the National Institute for Health and Care Excellence (NICE, 2018), and the Phoenix Australia Centre for Posttraumatic Mental Health (Phoenix Australia, 2013) converge on recommending trauma-focused cognitive behavioral therapies as the first-line intervention for PTSD. There are some medications with efficacy for treating PTSD, but the evidence for psychotherapy, and especially "trauma-focused" psychotherapy, is the strongest. Trauma-focused psychotherapies involve addressing the trauma directly, rather than just focusing on current symptoms and problems. Such approaches might involve examining thoughts about why the trauma happened, feeling emotions that match the facts of the trauma, confronting memories and reminders of the trauma, and/or narrating the story of the trauma, all with the purpose of processing the trauma so that one can recover from its effects. Thus, these therapies have in common not avoiding (a key maintaining factor in PTSD) but approaching the trauma memory so as to facilitate recovery. There are minor differences in the recommendations across guidelines as to the specific treatments recommended in each category, but the guidelines are more similar than different in their review of the evidence.

An example of the specific recommendations are those of VA/DoD. Their Clinical Practice Guideline for the Management of PTSD and Acute Stress Disorder provides guidance on intervention strategies with the strongest evidence. For the treatment of PTSD, VA/DoD (2023) guidelines recommend individual, manualized, trauma-focused psychotherapy over pharmacologic interventions. Specifically recommended with the greatest strength of evidence are prolonged exposure (PE), cognitive processing therapy (CPT), and eye movement desensitization and reprocessing (EMDR). Suggested with weaker evidence are cognitive therapy for PTSD (CT-PTSD), present-centered therapy (PCT), and written exposure therapy (WET). Because the VA/DoD guidelines are the most recently published, we will focus on describing and reviewing the evidence for the therapies "recommended" (strongest evidence) and "suggested" (less evidence but promising results) in these guidelines.

Although large differences have been observed in meta-analyses comparing first-line treatments to other, less effective interventions, studies that have been conducted to directly compare first-line, evidence-based PTSD treatments to one another have tended not to show significant differences (Resick et al., 2002; Sloan et al., 2018). While therapists often try to assign patients to the "right" treatment, research has shown that there are no consistent predictors of which patients will respond better to which evidence-based treatment at this time. Therefore, current best practices are to engage in *shared decision-making*, informing the patient about evidence-based treatment options and allowing patients to choose the specific PTSD treatment protocol that best suits them, among those with strong evidence. Addressing one's trauma is difficult work, so allowing the patient to select the evidence-based therapy that is most appealing to them may increase the chances that they complete treatment, which increases the chances of a good clinical outcome.

Overview of Evidence-Based Psychotherapies

As outlined above, the primary, recommended approach for the treatment of PTSD is cognitive behavioral therapy with a trauma focus. Within the category of cognitive behavioral therapy, there are a number of specific protocols that have been studied and accrued evidence supporting their efficacy (e.g., CPT, PE). These trauma-focused, cognitive behavioral therapies have much in common—for example, they all involve psychoeducation about PTSD and trauma recovery, encouragement not to avoid the trauma memory, and strategies to process the trauma. The specific strategies for trauma processing vary from protocol to protocol, with some protocols focusing more on behavioral interventions (e.g., exposure) and others focusing more on cognitive interventions (e.g., examining unhelpful beliefs).

Exposure-based therapies were originally developed to treat anxiety disorders, such as phobias. Because PTSD was originally categorized as an anxiety disorder, exposure-based therapies were developed and used to treat PTSD. Even though PTSD is no longer categorized among the anxiety disorders (now being in its own category of trauma- and stressor-related disorders), exposure continues to be a widely used and effective treatment approach for PTSD. Exposure for PTSD might include *imaginal exposure*—revisiting the trauma memory for the purpose of trauma processing—and/or *in vivo exposure*—confronting feared but safe situations "in real life". Specific protocols that use exposure include PE, WET, CT-PTSD, and narrative exposure therapy (NET).

Cognitive interventions are also used across a variety of disorders, such as anxiety and depressive disorders. They involve helping patients to identify thoughts or beliefs that may not be accurate or helpful and that lead to distressing emotions, and teaching patients skills to evaluate those thoughts and come up with more balanced, realistic thoughts. In the case of PTSD, trauma-focused cognitive interventions typically identify and address beliefs about the trauma itself (i.e., its cause, its consequences). Specific protocols that have a significant cognitive component include CPT and CT-PTSD.

Most evidence-based PTSD protocols include exposure, cognitive approaches, or a combination of both to different degrees. The two most widely studied PTSD treatments, which are recommended in all of the aforementioned clinical practice guidelines, are CPT and PE. Although PE emphasizes exposure more, whereas CPT focuses on cognitive strategies, both approaches result in new learning that helps patients recover from the effects of their traumas. A key feature across evidence-based, trauma-focused treatments is that they involve not avoiding the trauma memory but instead facing it in safe, therapeutic ways.

Prolonged Exposure

PE, developed by Foa et al. (2019) combines psychoeducation with the two types of exposure mentioned earlier: imaginal exposure and *in vivo* exposure. In PE, imaginal exposure involves having the patient recount the trauma aloud while revisiting it in their mind, followed by processing the experience. *In vivo* exposure involves gradually confronting situations that feel more dangerous since the trauma (but are objectively safe) as well as safe situations that are reminders of the trauma.

The treatment protocol for PE typically consists of 8–15 90-minute sessions, although 60-minute sessions have also been tested and shown to be no less effective (Foa et al., 2019; van Minnen & Foa, 2006). The first two sessions are devoted to information gathering, education about PTSD, explanations of the treatment rationale, treatment planning, and practicing breathing retraining. The remaining sessions focus on both imaginal and *in vivo* exposures. During the therapy sessions, patients are asked to close their eyes and to recount aloud what happened to them during the trauma in the present tense with as much detail as possible, including sensory details (e.g., sights, smells, sounds, sensations), as well as emotions and thoughts. Usually, the exposure is repeated two or three times in each session depending on the length of the account. Following the imaginal exposure, the therapist and patient process the experience. Sessions are audio recorded, and patients listen to the recording of the imaginal exposure each day between sessions. Patients also complete *in vivo* exposures. The therapist helps the patient to develop an *in vivo* hierarchy, and the patient works between sessions to gradually confront and stay in these safe situations that have been avoided since the trauma. During each exposure, patients track their distress levels using Subjective Unit of Discomfort Scale (SUDS) ratings ("On a scale from 0 to 100, how distressed are you?"). During initial exposures, anxiety is expected to be high. With repeated exposures in the safe therapy setting, anxiety typically diminishes, and patients also learn new information, including that they can tolerate the experience.

Marilyn sought treatment one year after an automobile accident that left her with chronic back and neck pain as well as PTSD. During a rainstorm, Marilyn was struck from the rear just after she came to a stop at a stoplight. Her car was forced into the car in front of her. Occasionally she had flashbacks of her accident, particularly on rainy days. She had occasional nightmares and expressed feelings of helplessness. Because of her injuries, Marilyn did not attempt to drive for several months following the accident. However, the longer she avoided, the more difficult it became to get back to driving, and she would end up calling a friend or coworker to give her a ride. Unfortunately, this approach wasn't practical because her friends weren't always available, so she sometimes had to miss work or pay high rates for a rideshare. It was her need for employment and the eroding of support from family and friends that brought her into treatment.

As per the PE protocol, treatment consisted of imaginal and in-vivo exposure. Although her re-experiencing symptoms and emotions regarding the accident diminished during the imaginal exposure, she continued to avoid driving due to fear she would have another accident. In order to help her with this avoidance, the therapist had Marilyn practice "driving" by first sitting in her car while it was parked in front of her house. Even just sitting in the car again was difficult because it brought up memories of the accident. Although she was initially quite anxious, Marilyn's fear diminished quickly, and she grew more comfortable. Gradually Marilyn began taking bigger steps, such as driving just around her block on fair weather days. As she developed more confidence in driving again, she continued to step up her exposure practice. Eventually she tackled the highest item on her list, driving in the rain in the area near where the accident happened. In the process of doing these exposures, Marilyn realized that while it is always possible to have an accident, she has been able to drive safely many times before and since the accident without issue. By the end of treatment, Marilyn was no longer reporting PTSD symptoms although she did report having some lingering tension on rainy days. She was not avoiding driving, however, and had not missed any work due to avoidance.

Research on PE

PE is one of the most studied therapies for PTSD, and dozens of clinical trials have been conducted demonstrating its efficacy. It is efficacious among civilians, veterans, and active duty service members, both when tested by the treatment developers and when tested by other research groups, lending additional support to the treatment's efficacy (e.g., Foa et al., 2022; Resick et al., 2002; Schnurr et al., 2022). In 2010, Powers and colleagues conducted a meta-analysis of randomized controlled trials (RCTs) of PE. PE demonstrated a large effect size and was superior to both active and inactive control conditions. It has also been shown to be effective in routine care settings (e.g., Eftekhari et al., 2013; Jacoby et al., 2022).

Building on the well-established efficacy and effectiveness of PE, researchers have studied strategies to understand its mechanisms so as to enhance its efficiency and implementation potential. Although PE was originally developed to include 45 minutes of imaginal exposure in 90-minute sessions, research has demonstrated that shorter intervals of imaginal exposure are effective, allowing PE to be delivered in 60-minute sessions, making it more portable to clinical settings (Foa et al., 2022). This is likely because research has also shown that between-session habituation (reductions in SUDS) is more important than within-session habituation in predicting outcome (Sripada & Rauch, 2015). Theorists have also better understood that improvement can occur even without habituation, as long as new learning occurs. Consistent with this theory, reductions in cognitive distortions decrease during PE and predict symptom outcome (Cooper et al., 2017).

Cognitive Processing Therapy

Resick and Schnicke (1993) developed CPT originally for use with rape and crime victims, CPT was adapted from cognitive therapy techniques explicated by Beck and Emery (1985). However, whereas Beckian cognitive therapy usually focuses on maladaptive beliefs about the present, CPT prioritizes beliefs about the trauma itself, such as why it happened and whether it could have been prevented. It is based on the theory that beliefs about the traumatic event might become distorted ("assimilation") in an attempt to maintain prior beliefs about oneself and the world. While "accommodation" of the new event into the person's belief system is desirable, "over-accommodation" (overgeneralization) may lead to extreme distortions about the safety or trustworthiness of others or overly harsh judgments about oneself (see Chapter 3 for more details). The therapist thus helps the patient examine whether the trauma appeared to disrupt or confirm beliefs prior to this experience and whether the patient has distorted the meaning of the event to fit with previous beliefs or overgeneralized (over-accommodated) from the event to their beliefs about themselves and the world. Patients are then taught to examine their own self-statements and to modify their extreme beliefs to bring them into balance.

CPT also places an emphasis on experiencing the "natural emotions" associated with the trauma—the universal, expected reactions that would result from danger, loss, and inflicted harm, which typically abate over time. However, "manufactured emotions" that are the product of distorted thinking (e.g., "I should have prevented the event" leading to guilt and shame) are addressed with primarily cognitive strategies throughout the therapy.

As research on CPT has advanced, changes have been made to the protocol. In the current standard version of CPT (Resick et al., 2024), treatment begins with a psychoeducation session in which the symptoms of PTSD are described and explained within cognitive theory. At the conclusion of that session, patients are asked to write about their thoughts about why the traumatic event occurred and what it means to them that the event happened. After reading and discussing this "impact statement" in Session 2 with an eye toward identifying problematic beliefs and cognitions ("stuck points"), patients are then taught to identify the connection between events, thoughts, and feelings and to practice at home with worksheets. Using a Socratic style of therapy, the therapist teaches patients to ask questions regarding their assumptions and self-statements to begin exploring them. Patients are taught to use worksheets to examine and replace maladaptive thoughts and beliefs. In the early stages of the therapy, the focus is typically on the patient's erroneous blame and attempts to undo the event after the fact (assimilation). In the final five sessions, the therapy progresses systematically through common areas of cognitive disruption: safety, trust, power/control, esteem, and intimacy. Originally CPT included writing an account of the traumatic event, but this is now an optional part of the CPT protocol, based on a study that showed that patients had just as much symptom improvement in CPT without the written accounts (Resick et al., 2008). CPT was originally developed as 12 sessions, but can be variable length, based on patient response (Galovski et al., 2012; Resick et al., 2021).

After going to a movie one night, David was assaulted by two young men in a dark parking lot. They asked him for money. When he refused, one of the young men pulled out a knife. David swore at them and turned to run. The young man with the knife suddenly lunged at him and stabbed him in the shoulder. The two men ran away after grabbing his wallet. Two years after the incident, David was referred to therapy by his sister who was concerned because he seemed depressed.

The therapist diagnosed both PTSD and depression. In addition to the assault, David reported that as a child he had been physically and emotionally abused by his father, who had an alcohol use disorder. Although David had never drank much alcohol in the past, he found himself drinking in the evening, particularly before going to bed. He expressed fear of becoming

*like his father. CPT was implemented. When David wrote his impact state-
ment about the meaning of the event, it became clear that David was har-
boring a great deal of self-blame for the incident. He kept playing over in
his mind ways he could have handled the situation differently or more hero-
ically. It was also evident that he was fearful of going out, was ashamed
that he was fearful, and had begun judging himself harshly in many ways.
David was afraid that if others knew how he felt, they would ridicule or
reject him. As a result, he withdrew socially and became more and more
depressed.*

*David learned to examine his self-blame about the crime through
Socratic questioning by the therapist and a series of worksheets he completed between sessions. He came to realize that blame belonged to the
assailants, not to him, and that their behavior was not predictable or
controllable by his actions or inactions. He also realized that he had been
assuming other people were all sharing his harsh self-judgments; that he
had been "mind reading" rather than finding out what the people in his life
actually thought. Through the therapy, David began to identify negative
patterns of thinking that predated the assault and probably resulted from
the childhood abuse. He was able to re-examine these beliefs, not only with
regard to the assault, but the child abuse as well. As he began to reassess
his thoughts and assumptions and replace them with more balanced beliefs,
his PTSD symptoms and depression began to lift and he had less desire to
drink. David began to reconnect with friends and family and was able to
resume going out without difficulty.*

Research on CPT

Like PE, dozens of RCTs have demonstrated the efficacy of CPT for PTSD, and
numerous meta-analyses have shown large effect sizes for CPT (e.g., Watts et al.,
2013). CPT has been shown to work with civilians, veterans, and active duty service
members when examined by the treatment developers as well as outside research
teams (Butollo et al., 2015; Forbes et al., 2012; Peterson et al., 2022; Resick et al.,
2002), in traditional therapeutic settings, via telehealth (Morland et al., 2020), as well
as in low-resource settings (Bass et al., 2013). In a meta-analysis of CPT studies,
Asmundson et al. (2019) determined that CPT demonstrated superiority over inactive
controls with large effect sizes and was superior to active controls at posttreatment
though not different at follow-up.

Like PE, researchers have built on the strong empirical foundation of CPT's efficacy and effectiveness and examined approaches to enhance CPT's efficiency and
precision. CPT has been adapted cross-culturally and delivered successfully in many

countries including Germany, Australia, Japan, Iraq, and the Democratic Republic of Congo (Bass et al., 2013; Forbes et al., 2012; Kaysen et al., 2013; Pearson et al., 2019; Takagishi et al., 2023). Because CPT works both with and without a written account of the trauma (Resick et al., 2008), either version is effective and recommended in clinical practice guidelines (VA/DoD, 2023). When flexing the length of treatment as part of a variable-length approach (e.g., extending the treatment for a limited number of additional sessions), even more patients are categorized as responders (reaching subthreshold or a low symptom level) rather than nonresponders (Galovski et al., 2012; Resick et al., 2021).

Eye Movement Desensitization and Reprocessing

EMDR is a controversial therapy that evolved from a personal observation by the treatment developer (Shapiro, 1989, 2018) that troubling thoughts were resolved when following the waving of leaves during a walk in the park. Shapiro developed EMDR on the basis of this observation and argued that lateral eye movements facilitate cognitive processing of the trauma. EMDR is now described as an eight-phase treatment that includes history taking, patient preparation, target assessment, desensitization, installation, body scan, closure, and reevaluation of treatment effects. EMDR includes both exposure and cognitive components as well as the lateral eye movements.

In the EMDR protocol, a patient is asked to identify and focus on a traumatic image or memory (target assessment phase). Next, the therapist elicits negative belief statements about the memory. The patient is asked to assign a rating to the memory and negative beliefs on an 11-point scale of distress and to identify the physical location of the anxiety. The therapist helps the patient generate positive thoughts that would be preferable to associate with the memory. These are rated on a 7-point scale of how much the patient believes the statement. Once the therapist has instructed the patient in the basic EMDR procedure, the patient is asked to do four things simultaneously (desensitization phase): (1) visualize the memory, (2) rehearse the negative thoughts, (3) concentrate on the physical sensations of the anxiety, and (4) visually track the therapist's index finger. While the patient does this, the therapist rapidly moves their index finger back and forth 30–35 cm from the patient's face, with two back-and-forth movements per second. These are repeated 24 times. Then the patient is asked to blank out the memory and take a deep breath. Subsequently, the patient brings back the memory and thoughts and rates the level of distress. Sets of eye movements are repeated until the distress rating equals 0 or 1. At this point, the patient describes how they feel about the positive cognition and gives a rating for it (installation phase).

Research on EMDR

Although Shapiro maintains that lateral eye movements are an essential therapeutic component of EMDR, studies that have examined this have found mixed results. Renfrey and Spates (1994) treated a sample of 23 trauma victims with standard EMDR, or one of two variations including one condition in which no lateral eye movements were induced and subjects were instructed to fix their visual attention. All three groups improved significantly on measures of PTSD, depression, anxiety, heart rate, and subjective distress scores, and no differences were found among treatments. Devilly and colleagues (1998) compared EMDR to two control conditions with Vietnam veterans in Australia. One of the control conditions was identical to EMDR except for the eye movements. Instead of lateral eye movements, patients were asked to fix their gaze on a black box that emitted a flashing light while imagining the trauma. The other control condition was treatment as usual from their therapists. Devilly et al. found that both of the treatment groups improved somewhat compared to the treatment as usual group, but the two experimental groups did not differ statistically. At a six-month follow-up, the treatment gains were not maintained for either experimental group.

It does not appear that lateral eye movements are an essential component of EMDR. EMDR forces the patient to think about the trauma, to identify the negative cognitions associated with the trauma, and to work toward positive cognitions as they process the traumatic memory. Without the lateral eye movements, EMDR is quite similar to other forms of cognitive/exposure therapy that facilitate the processing of the traumatic memory. Therefore, any efficacy demonstrated by EMDR may be more attributable to engagement of the traumatic memory and the facilitation of information processing than to eye movements.

Overall, clinical trials have demonstrated that EMDR is effective at reducing PTSD symptoms and performs well, particularly when compared to no treatment and nonexposure therapies (Davidson & Parker, 2001). There has been mixed evidence and conclusions about the efficacy of EMDR relative to other treatments in meta-analyses. Some meta-analyses have shown that EMDR was slightly more effective than cognitive behavioral therapy (Chen et al., 2015), while other more recent meta-analyses have shown the opposite pattern of results. For example, one meta-analysis found that CPT was twice as effective as EMDR (Jericho et al., 2022). It should be noted that randomized, controlled head-to-head comparison trials are better for determining the comparative effectiveness of interventions because they overcome the interpretative challenges of differing populations, methods, and other factors between trials. EMDR appears to be efficacious in treating PTSD, but owing to the mixed state of the literature, as well as lack of clarity about the treatment mechanisms, EMDR is recommended as a first-line treatment in some clinical practice guidelines (ISTSS, Phoenix Australia, NICE) but suggested with more temperance by other organizations (VA/DoD, APA).

Written Exposure Therapy

Sloan and Marx (2019) developed a five-session, exposure-based therapy (WET) in which individuals repeatedly write about their trauma to facilitate trauma recovery. It was developed based on Pennebaker and Beall's (1986) written disclosure procedure but adapted to also include psychoeducation, a treatment rationale, and a greater dose of exposure via more writing sessions. Patients write about their most traumatic experience for 30 minutes in each session in response to specific prompts. In the first three sessions, the participant is prompted to write in detail about the trauma, including thoughts and feelings experienced during the event. The remaining sessions also include a focus on the impact of the event on their lives. The therapist engages the patient prior to writing to check-in on how things went between sessions and to give feedback on how well the prompt was followed at the previous session. After the writing, the therapist also briefly engages with the patient to discuss the experience of writing. However, overall, the amount of interaction with the therapist is less in WET than in treatments like PE and CPT. Patients receiving WET are encouraged to allow themselves to think about the trauma between sessions, but no formal between session practice is assigned. WET is theorized to work via exposure and overcoming avoidance, which allows for trauma processing to occur.

Research on WET

WET is a newer treatment protocol but has been accruing evidence in recent years. In clinical trials, WET has been efficacious with civilians, veterans, and active duty service members (Sloan et al., 2012, 2013, 2018, 2022, 2023). In a pilot study, 86% of veterans receiving WET had a clinically significant decrease in PTSD symptoms by the three-month follow-up (Sloan et al., 2013). In the first RCT of WET, adults with PTSD from a motor vehicle accident had significant reductions in PTSD symptoms, with 100% exhibiting a reliable change, and large between-group effect sizes compared to waitlist (Sloan et al., 2012). After determining WET's initial efficacy, the treatment developers began comparing WET to first-line treatment approaches using a non-inferiority design, which tests whether differences between treatment arms are within a predetermined margin that would suggest WET is no less effective than the comparison treatment. The first of these non-inferiority RCTs compared WET to CPT+A (CPT with the trauma account) among veterans and civilians. WET was non-inferior to CPT+A on PTSD symptom improvement (Sloan et al., 2018), and treatment gains were maintained for both treatments for 60 weeks post the first treatment session (Thompson-Hollands et al., 2018). In another non-inferiority design, WET was also non-inferior to CPT (without the trauma accounts) among active duty service members (Sloan et al., 2022). Finally, WET was compared to PE, and also was shown to be non-inferior (Sloan et al., 2023).

WET has also been shown to be tolerable and satisfactory to patients, with low dropout, typically ranging from 6% to 14% (Sloan et al., 2012, 2013, 2018). In the non-inferiority trial, significantly fewer patients dropped out of WET (6%) compared to CPT (39%; Sloan et al., 2018). In the trial of WET among active duty service members, a higher dropout rate was observed of about 25%, but dropout tends to be high among active duty military. It appears that WET has particularly low dropout when delivered via telehealth (LoSavio et al., 2023; Sloan et al., 2023). In a meta-analysis, WET had significantly lower dropout than other treatments (Jericho et al., 2022), which is encouraging given that dropout from trauma-focused treatments can serve as a barrier to receiving an adequate dose and benefitting from care. The emerging research on WET is promising, although to date it has been conducted primarily by the treatment developers, so additional studies by other research groups will be important.

Other Written Narrative Therapies

WET is part of a class of therapies involving narrative writing. Another notable therapy in this category is NET (Schauer et al., 2011). In the VA/DoD (2023) guidelines, the recommendation was "neither for nor against" NET based on insufficient evidence, namely mixed results from studies comparing NET to active treatments. However, the NICE (2018) guidelines do recommend NET. NET has been studied more in Europe than in the United States and has been most commonly implemented with refugee populations. It involves providing a chronological narration of one's entire life, with a focus on traumatic experiences, facilitated by a therapist (see Robjant & Fazel, 2010). NET has been well studied, including in open trials and RCTs, and compared to waitlist, psychoeducation, treatment as usual, meditation/relaxation, supportive counseling, or other active treatments (Robjant & Fazel, 2010; Sloan et al., 2015). In a recent meta-analysis of 16 RCTs, NET was superior to non-active comparison conditions as well as non-trauma-focused treatments (Lely et al., 2019).

Cognitive Therapy for PTSD

CT-PTSD is a specific protocol for PTSD based on Ehlers and Clark's (2000) cognitive model of PTSD. Compared to the previously mentioned protocols, the CT-PTSD protocol is more flexible, involving the selection of cognitive and behavioral interventions for PTSD, consistent with cognitive behavioral therapy for other disorders. CT-PTSD includes both cognitive and behavioral approaches such as exposure and cognitive restructuring.

Core interventions in CT-PTSD are as follows: (1) developing an individualized case formulation; (2) guiding the patient to complete reclaiming/rebuilding your life assignments (i.e., to reclaim meaningful activities and social contacts); (3) changing problematic trauma-related appraisals (i.e., personal meanings) through guided discovery, behavioral experiments, etc.; (4) using imaginal or narrative writing combined with reflection to update trauma memories; (5) exposure discrimination training to help differentiate triggers "now" versus the trauma "then"; (6) a physical or virtual visit to the site of the trauma; (7) dropping unhelpful behaviors and cognitive processes (e.g., rumination, hypervigilance); and (8) developing a blueprint summarizing what the patient has learned and planning for the future (Ehlers et al., 2005). Though these are the core elements of CT-PTSD, there is flexibility in the selection and delivery of the specific strategies.

Research on CT-PTSD

CT-PTSD has been shown to be efficacious across a small number of clinical trials. In the first of these (Ehlers et al., 2003), motor vehicle accident survivors were randomized to receive CT-PTSD, a self-help booklet based on cognitive behavioral therapy, or repeated assessments. CT-PTSD was superior to both other conditions, and only 11% had PTSD post-intervention, compared to 61% and 55% in the self-help and assessment conditions, respectively. Ehlers et al. (2005) randomized community patients to waitlist or CT-PTSD, comprising up to 12 weekly, 60–90-minute sessions. There were large effect sizes, with those receiving CT-PTSD improving on PTSD, depression, anxiety, and other outcomes, with 79% of patients remitting from PTSD. Impressively there were no dropouts from CT-PTSD in either trial. Ehlers et al. (2014) conducted an RCT to compare a seven-day intensive CT-PTSD, a standard CT-PTSD, an emotion-focused supportive therapy, and a wait list group. At post-treatment, more than three quarters of participants receiving CT-PTSD, 43% of the emotion-focused treatment, and 7% of the waitlist had recovered from PTSD. CT-PTSD also demonstrated large effect sizes when delivered as part of an RCT in community centers in Northern Ireland for individuals with PTSD, mostly secondary to terrorism and other civil conflict. CT-PTSD has not been as widely studied or implemented as CPT or PE, and has not been studied by independent groups, but it appears to be a promising example of effective trauma-focused cognitve behavioral therapy.

Present-Centered Therapy

PCT is unique on this list in that it is a non-trauma-focused treatment and does not involve approaching the trauma memory specifically. It was originally developed as an active control condition for clinical trials of PTSD psychotherapy to account for the nonspecifics of therapy such as time and attention, but it has performed well and thus is a viable treatment option for individuals with PTSD. PCT involves psychoeducation about PTSD and the relationship between PTSD and current problems and teaches problem-solving to address current problems and symptoms. Patients complete daily diaries to monitor problems, symptoms, and stressors that occur during the week. In session, the therapist helps the patient identify a problem that they would like to focus on, and they work collaboratively to develop possible solutions to try over the next week. Therapists do not direct patients to engage in exposure or cognitive restructuring, but if patients independently identify that approaching situations or reexamining their thoughts might be helpful, they may do so.

Research on PCT

Schnurr and colleagues (2003) compared group-administered PCT to trauma-focused group therapy among Vietnam-era veterans. Both groups improved, and there was no difference between groups in PTSD in the intent-to-treat sample, though there was less dropout from PCT. Among treatment completers, the trauma-focused treatment showed an advantage on some PTSD symptom clusters. McDonagh et al. (2005) compared PCT to cognitive behavioral therapy (imaginal and *in vivo* exposure, breathing retraining, and cognitive restructuring) and a waitlist control among women with PTSD who had experienced childhood sexual abuse. Both treatments were superior to waitlist. Again, among the intent-to-treat sample, there were no differences between treatments, but there was less dropout from PCT. Among completers only, there were fewer participants who met criteria for PTSD at follow-up in the cognitive behavioral therapy group. Among female veterans and active duty military, PE was superior to PCT, though both treatments resulted in reductions in PTSD (Schnurr et al., 2007). Differences between treatments were more modest at later follow-ups. Again there was an advantage for PCT in retention of patients.

Classen et al. (2011) compared group PCT to trauma-focused group therapy and a waitlist control group among adult survivors of childhood sexual abuse who were at risk for human immunodeficiency virus (HIV) infection due to risky sexual behavior and substance use. There were no differences between PCT and trauma-focused group therapy on PTSD, but PCT had an advantage for HIV risk, whereas trauma-focused group therapy had an advantage for anger/irritability. In another study, Surís and colleagues (2013) compared PCT to CPT among veterans with PTSD from military sexual trauma. Again, both treatments showed large effects. Posttreatment, there were no differences between PCT and CPT on depression or a clinician-administered PTSD scale, but outcomes were better for CPT on self-reported PTSD symptoms. Resick et al. (2015) compared group CPT to group PCT and found that both interventions led to large reductions in PTSD, though improvement was greater in CPT, and CPT was more effective at addressing depression.

Overall, research has demonstrated that even without specific trauma-focused components, PCT typically performs well compared to even first-line trauma-focused interventions. It may be that the lower dropout in PCT contributes to the positive outcomes observed. Nonetheless, while not recommended in any clinical practice guidelines as a first-choice treatment, it is noted in some guidelines (VA/DoD, 2023) as a suggested option with some evidence for its use.

Pharmacological Treatments

As noted earlier, psychopharmacological intervention is not the first-line recommended treatment for PTSD. However, medication is frequently offered by primary care physicians and psychiatrists to deal with some of the symptoms that are problematic for trauma survivors. Psychopharmacological treatments are also recommended if individual psychotherapy is not available or not preferred by the patient (VA/DoD, 2023). Furthermore, APA (2017) concluded that comparative effectiveness for pharmacological versus psychotherapeutic interventions could not be concluded based on the evidence and that additional research is needed.

In some cases, medication may help to relieve the severity of symptoms and may allow the affected person to sleep and to function, or to engage in trauma-focused psychotherapy. However, if the trauma survivor is using the medication to avoid dealing with the trauma memory, it is likely that these symptoms will reemerge when the medication is discontinued. Medications also have a number of side effects that may be troublesome.

Among psychopharmacological interventions, antidepressant medications have the most support for PTSD. VA/DoD (2023) clinical practice guidelines indicate that the evidence for treating PTSD is strongest for paroxetine, sertraline, and venlafaxine. APA (2017) and ISTSS (2018) guidelines also recommend fluoxetine. These recommendations are consistent with guidance, across clinical practice guidelines, that while psychopharmacological interventions have a weaker strength of evidence compared to trauma-focused psychotherapy, selective serotonin reuptake inhibitors (SSRIs) are among the most supported pharmacological interventions for PTSD.

Several other medications were categorized as having insufficient evidence for or against their use for PTSD (e.g., bupropion, citalopram, duloxetine, fluoxetine, imipramine, mirtazapine, topiramate, quetiapine). Other medications have evidence *against* their use (e.g., ketamine, prazosin, risperidone), and one class of medications that is consistently noted to be contraindicated for PTSD (i.e., strong evidence against its use) is benzodiazepines (e.g., Xanax, Valium). In a meta-analysis, benzodiazepines were summarized to be not only ineffective for PTSD but also associated with significant risks including worse functioning and therapeutic outcomes (Guina et al., 2015).

Psychotherapy for PTSD and Comorbid Disorders

An evolving area of study is how best to treat PTSD when it occurs in the presence of other, comorbid disorders. Studies, most focused on CPT and PE, have demonstrated that these first-line, trauma-focused treatments are not only effective when there are comorbid conditions, but that typically symptoms of the comorbid disorder improve as well. This is the case for depression symptoms, suicidal ideation, alcohol misuse, and even personality disorders (Bovin et al., 2017; Brown et al., 2019; Bryan et al., 2016; Dondanville et al., 2019; Resick et al., 2002). When patients have a more "complex" presentation, such as childhood as well as adult traumas and more emotional dysregulation, some have raised the question of whether a "phase-based" approach is needed, with skills training prior to addressing the trauma; however, research on phase-based approaches has failed to demonstrate an advantage over trauma-focused treatments alone (De Jongh et al., 2016). In the VA/DoD (2023) clinical practice guidelines, there was not sufficient evidence to recommend for or against phase-based treatment like Skills Training in Affective and Interpersonal Regulation (STAIR; Cloitre et al., 2002).

Although there is now ample evidence that PTSD can be treated in the context of comorbid issues, nonetheless, clinicians must conceptualize their patients and develop a treatment plan including which problems to address and in what order. Historically, it was commonly the case that mental disorders were conceptualized as separate issues and treated individually. However, it is now more common to consider commonalities and shared mechanisms of psychological disorders. Researchers have been examining combinations of interventions and testing their sequence to determine what might be most effective. For example, researchers have tested intervention packages combining CPT with behavioral activation (an intervention involving scheduling activities that bring a sense of mastery or pleasure) for depression, cognitive behavioral therapy for insomnia, smoking counseling, and compensatory cognitive training for traumatic brain injury (Angelakis et al., 2020; Jak et al., 2019; Taylor et al., 2023; Wells et al., 2022). Likewise, researchers have tested PE combined with dialectical behavior therapy (a therapy focused on developing skills related to distress tolerance, emotion regulation, interpersonal effectiveness, and mindfulness) and substance use treatment (Back et al., 2014; Harned et al., 2021).

In the case of substance use disorders, for many years PTSD and substance use were treated sequentially, and trauma and PTSD would often be approached last. Individuals with PTSD and comorbid substance use disorders may have even had to obtain some extended period of continuous abstinence before being offered a trauma-focused treatment (if ever). However, current guidelines recommend combined or concurrent treatment of PTSD and substance use disorders. As such, researchers have been testing protocols that combine evidence-based treatments, such as Concurrent Treatment of PTSD and Substance Use Disorders Using Prolonged Exposure (COPE; Back et al., 2014). Each of the treatment combinations discussed in this section need more research; however, it is important to note that PTSD can be addressed even in the context of comorbid conditions and that innovative research is underway to determine optimal strategies for effectively and efficiently addressing multiple disorders.

Treatment of Other Trauma- and Stressor-Related Disorders

Compared to the literature on treatments for PTSD, there is an extremely limited amount of research on treatments for other trauma- and stressor-related disorders. Following is a summary of the literature on the two most studied trauma- and stressor-related disorders after PTSD: acute stress disorder and adjustment disorder.

Part of the challenge of studying treatment for acute stress disorder and adjustment disorder is that, by definition, these disorders are brief in their duration/chronicity. Thus, there is a narrow window of time during which to study people before they recover or are diagnosed with something else, such as PTSD. If clinicians initially offer lower intensity psychological interventions, stepping up to a more intensive intervention may be indicated if symptoms persist or worsen (Domhardt & Baumeister, 2018).

Acute Stress Disorder

In addition to PTSD, the VA/DoD (2023) clinical practice guidelines also discuss treatment recommendations for acute stress disorder. Recommended are individual, manualized, trauma-focused, brief, cognitive behavioral therapy, as well as collaborative care; wellness-oriented activities; education; normalization; acute symptom management; social support; and continued assessment to determine if symptoms persist and become PTSD.

In an early treatment study, Bryant et al. (1998) compared cognitive behavioral therapy for acute stress disorder to supportive counseling and found that only 8% of patients met criteria for PTSD at posttreatment compared to 83% of those who received supportive counseling. In another RCT, researchers compared five sessions of exposure (imaginal and *in vivo*) to five sessions of cognitive restructuring and a waitlist control condition. Those in the exposure condition fared best: After treatment, only 33% of patients in the exposure treatment met criteria for PTSD compared to 63% of those who received cognitive structuring and 77% who were in the waitlist condition (Bryant et al., 2008). This suggests that, as stand-alone interventions, exposure may be more helpful in the initial aftermath of trauma.

Across two RCTs, Nixon (2012; Nixon et al., 2016) examined the effects of CPT compared to active control treatments among individuals with acute stress disorder. In the first study (Nixon, 2012), recent survivors of interpersonal assault improved on depression and PTSD symptoms during CPT or supportive counseling, with statistically nonsignificant, moderate-to-large effect sizes favoring CPT. Comparing CPT and treatment as usual among survivors of sexual assault with acute stress disorder, Nixon and colleagues (2016) again observed that both groups reduced PTSD and depression symptoms, with no statistically significant differences, possibly due to the small sample size, but generally larger effect sizes, more clients reaching a good end-state of functioning, and less posttreatment service utilization seen among those receiving CPT. These studies suggest that evidence-based PTSD treatment protocols like CPT might be useful as early intervention for those with acute stress disorder in the wake of trauma.

Adjustment Disorder

Despite how commonly adjustment disorder is diagnosed, there has been a paucity of research on the most effective treatment for it. Conducting a review of the literature on psychological interventions for adjustment disorder, Domhardt and Baumeister (2018) found 33 studies—17 of which were RCTs and the other 16 of which were pilot or case studies. The authors summarized that interventions for adjustment disorder tended to have in common a focus on efforts to (1) reduce the impact of or remove the stressor, (2) enhance coping, and/or (3) invoke behavioral change to improve functioning.

Low-intensity interventions such as self-help, support groups, mindfulness/relaxation, behavioral activation, and e-health interventions have been tested for adjustment disorder. For example, in one RCT, burglary victims with full or subthreshold adjustment disorder had greater improvement in symptoms if they received a cognitive behavioral self-help protocol compared to waitlist (Bachem & Maercker, 2016). In an RCT of mindfulness training, participants with adjustment disorder exhibited improvements in psychological symptoms and quality of life (Bos et al., 2014). The evidence for cognitive behavioral therapy has been relatively weak for adjustment disorder, compared to its strength for other disorders, at least when examining functional outcomes like returning to work (Arends et al., 2012).

In a systematic review of therapy for adjustment disorder, O'Donnell et al. (2018) identified 29 studies (12 RCTs) focused on psychological (59%) and pharmacological (35%) treatments, with studies assessing a wide range of interventions (e.g., psychodynamic therapy, bibliotherapy, cognitive behavioral therapy), many using uncontrolled designs. Importantly, the quality of the studies was graded as "low" to "very low", limiting confidence in any study findings. Numerous methodological issues hamper interpretation of the study findings, including small sample sizes, inconsistent and nonspecific measurement strategies, lack of follow-up measures, and limited reporting of outcomes, among other issues.

A weakness of the literature on adjustment disorder interventions is that samples are often comprised of participants with a mixture of diagnoses including adjustment disorder, depression, or anxiety disorders. There are also a number of subtypes of adjustment disorder (APA, 2013), and it is unclear if there is heterogeneity in treatment response based on subtype. Overall, the quality of evidence for research on adjustment disorder treatments has been low, so optimal treatment is not well understood.

Prolonged Grief Disorder

In spite of the fact that prolonged grief disorder is new in the DSM-5, there have been many RCTs in its earlier iterations such as complicated grief (Shear, 2015). Complicated grief treatment studies have components to help the patient discuss the nature of loss and adaptation, promoting self-regulation, reappraising troubling thoughts and beliefs, "dosing" emotional pain (confront and set aside), building connections with others, setting goals to encourage hope and positive emotions, revisiting avoidance, and recounting the story of the death to create an acceptable account. Some other studies have examined more typical cognitive behavioral treatments (Bryant et al., 2014) that have also been found helpful. The Bryant et al. study compared cognitive behavioral therapy alone versus with exposure and found that adding exposure led to greater decreases in depression, negative appraisals, and functional impairment, as well as criteria for prolonged grief. Szuhany et al. (2021) reviewed both specific complicated grief treatments and cognitive behavioral therapy that includes cognitive restructuring and exposure and found them to be effective in reducing symptoms. In a meta-analysis of complicated grief treatment compared to various treatments as usual, Wittouck et al. (2011) found the complicated grief treatment to be superior.

Future Directions

Treatment research, especially for PTSD, is continuing to advance. A number of existing treatments are effective, and the majority of patients who complete them are able to recover from PTSD and other disabling symptoms. However, treatment dropout remains high, and the reach of these treatments to patients in care settings is low. Hopefully, the next decade of research will continue to make treatments more efficient and tolerable and produce even higher response rates. Additionally, while a number of evidence-based models are now available to treat PTSD and comorbid issues, and these models tend to work for people overall, research is needed to better determine what works best for whom and under what conditions to optimize and tailor treatment to the individual.

Researchers are also examining novel applications of existing interventions, such as mobile and massed versions of treatments (i.e., sessions spaced closer together, such as daily instead of weekly; Foa et al., 2018; Held et al., 2022; McLean et al., 2021), which appears to reduce dropout. Researchers are also focusing on common comorbidities and exploring treatments that combine interventions for different disorders, such as treatment for PTSD with treatment for sleep, pain, or substance use, as well as the optimal sequence of such interventions. Undoubtedly, the next decade of research will produce new innovations in treatment development.

Research on trauma- and stressor-related disorders other than PTSD has lagged behind the PTSD literature. Greater diagnostic clarity and larger and higher quality studies are needed to inform the way forward for patients with these diagnoses.

Summary

This chapter reviewed the most research-supported therapies that are based on theories of why people develop and get stuck with problematic symptoms after trauma. Psychotherapy, particularly cognitive behavioral therapy with a trauma focus, has the most evidence for successfully treating PTSD. To date, no one treatment has been shown to be more effective overall than the others, though CPT and PE are the most well-studied and most consistently recommended in clinical practice guidelines. Although medication is not recommended as the first-line approach for PTSD or other trauma- and stressor-related disorders, there are medications such as SSRIs that may provide relief.

Each of the psychotherapies discussed in this chapter is a treatment package consisting of various components, some of which are similar across treatments. In other words, because all of the treatments may involve these elements to some degree (psychoeducation, strategies to stop avoiding and process the trauma), it appears that there are multiple pathways to trauma recovery including through exposure and/or cognitive approaches. Resick and Schnicke (1993) have noted that one reason that so many treatment comparison studies for PTSD have not found differences among treatments may be due to the fact that almost all of the treatments include, either formally or informally, corrective information that may facilitate information processing.

Clinicians commonly inquire whether patients can be matched to the treatment that will be most effective for them. Despite efforts to identify predictors of treatment outcome, there are no clear and consistent findings to date indicating in advance which patients will benefit most from which treatment. Because multiple evidence-based treatments have been developed and found effective, shared decision-making about the specific evidence-based treatment that a patient would like to pursue is recommended. High dropout rates from trauma-focused treatments suggest that having a patient bought-in and motivated to complete a given treatment is important and is likely to increase the odds that they receive an adequate dose and benefit from the intervention.

References

American Psychiatric Association (APA) (2013). *Diagnostic and statistical manual of mental disorders* (5th ed.; DSM-5). Washington, D.C.: American Psychiatric Association.

American Psychological Association (APA). (2017). Clinical practice guideline for the treatment of posttraumatic stress disorder (PTSD) in adults. Retrieved from https://www.apa.org/ptsd-guideline/ptsd.pdf

Angelakis, S., Weber, N., & Nixon, R. D. (2020). Comorbid posttraumatic stress disorder and major depressive disorder: The usefulness of a sequential treatment approach within a randomised design. *Journal of Anxiety Disorders, 76*, 102324.

Arends, I., Bruinvels, D. J., Rebergen, D. S., Nieuwenhuijsen, K., Madan, I., Neumeyer-Gromen, A., Bultmann, U., & Verbeek, J. H. (2012). Interventions to facilitate return to work in adults with adjustment disorders. *Cochrane Database of Systematic Reviews, 12* (12), Art. No CD006389-. Article 006389.

Asmundson, G. J., Thorisdottir, A. S., Roden-Foreman, J. W., Baird, S. O., Witcraft, S. M., Stein, A. T., Smits, J. A., & Powers, M. B. (2019). A meta-analytic review of cognitive processing therapy for adults with posttraumatic stress disorder. *Cognitive Behaviour Therapy, 48*(1), 1–14.

Bachem, R., & Maercker, A. (2016). Self-help interventions for adjustment disorder problems: A randomized waiting-list controlled study in a sample of burglary victims. *Cognitive Behaviour Therapy, 45*(5), 397–413.

Back, S. E., Killeen, T. K., Cotton, B. D., & Carroll, K. M. (2014). *Concurrent treatment of PTSD and substance use disorders using prolonged exposure (COPE): Therapist guide.* New York: Oxford University Press.

Bass, J. K., Annan, J., McIvor Murray, S., Kaysen, D., Griffiths, S., Cetinoglu, T., Wachter, K., Murray, L. K., & Bolton, P. A. (2013). Controlled trial of psychotherapy for Congolese survivors of sexual violence. *New England Journal of Medicine, 368*(23), 2182–2191.

Beck, A. T., & Emery, G. (1985). *Anxiety disorders and phobias: A cognitive perspective.* New York: Basic Books.

Bos, E. H., Merea, R., van den Brink, E., Sanderman, R., & Bartels-Velthuis, A. A. (2014). Mindfulness training in a heterogeneous psychiatric sample: Outcome evaluation and comparison of different diagnostic groups. *Journal of Clinical Psychology, 70*(1), 60–71.

Bovin, M. J., Wolf, E. J., & Resick, P. A. (2017). Longitudinal associations between posttraumatic stress disorder severity and personality disorder features among female rape survivors. *Frontiers in Psychiatry, 8*, 240379.

Brown, L. A., McLean, C. P., Zang, Y., Zandberg, L., Mintz, J., Yarvis, J. S., Litz, B. T., Peterson, A. L., Bryan, C. J., Fina, B., Petersen, J., Dondanville, K. A., Roache, J. D., Young-McCaughan, S., & Foa, E. B. (2019). Does prolonged exposure increase suicide risk? Results from an active duty military sample. *Behaviour Research and Therapy, 118*, 87–93.

Bryan, C. J., Clemans, T. A., Hernandez, A. M., Mintz, J., Peterson, A. L., Yarvis, J. S., Resick, P. A., & The STRONG STAR Consortium. (2016). Evaluating potential iatrogenic suicide risk in trauma-focused group cognitive behavioral therapy for the treatment of PTSD in active duty military personnel. *Depression and Anxiety, 33*(6), 549–557.

Bryant, R. A., Harvey, A. G., Dang, S. T., Sackville, T., & Basten, C. (1998). Treatment of acute stress disorder: A comparison of cognitive-behavioral therapy and supportive counseling. *Journal of Consulting and Clinical Psychology, 66*(5), 862–866.

Bryant, R. A., Kenny, L., Joscelyne, A., Rawson, N., Maccallum, F., Cahill, C., Hopwood, S., Aderka, I., & Nickerson, A. (2014). Treating prolonged grief disorder: A randomized clinical trial. *JAMA Psychiatry, 71*, 1332–1339.

Bryant, R. A., Mastrodomenico, J., Felmingham, K. L., Hopwood, S., Kenny, L., Kandris, E., Cahill, C., & Creamer, M. (2008). Treatment of acute stress disorder: A randomized controlled trial. *Archives of General Psychiatry, 65*(6), 659–667.

Butollo, W., Karl, R., König, J., & Rosner, R. (2015). A randomized controlled clinical trial of dialogical exposure therapy vs. cognitive processing therapy for adult outpatients suffering from PTSD after type I trauma in adulthood. *Psychotherapy and Psychosomatics, 85*, 16–26.

Chen, L., Zhang, G., Hu, M., & Liang, X. (2015). Eye movement desensitization and reprocessing versus cognitive-behavioral therapy for adult posttraumatic stress disorder: Systematic review and meta-analysis. *The Journal of Nervous and Mental Disease, 203*(6), 443–451.

Classen, C. C., Palesh, O. G., Cavanaugh, C. E., Koopman, C., Kaupp, J. W., Kraemer, H. C., Aggarwal, R., & Spiegel, D. (2011). A comparison of trauma-focused and present-focused group therapy for survivors of childhood sexual abuse: A randomized controlled trial. *Psychological Trauma: Theory, Research, Practice, and Policy, 3*(1), 84–93.

Cloitre, M., Koenen, K. C., Cohen, L. R., & Han, H. (2002). Skills training in affective and interpersonal regulation followed by exposure: A phase-based treatment for PTSD related to childhood abuse. *Journal of Consulting and Clinical Psychology, 70*(5), 1067–1074.

Cooper, A. A., Zoellner, L. A., Roy-Byrne, P., Mavissakalian, M. R., & Feeny, N. C. (2017). Do changes in trauma-related beliefs predict PTSD symptom improvement in prolonged exposure and sertraline? *Journal of Consulting and Clinical Psychology, 85*(9), 873–882.

Davidson, P. R., & Parker, K. C. (2001). Eye movement desensitization and reprocessing (EMDR): A meta-analysis. *Journal of Consulting and Clinical Psychology, 69*(2), 305–316.

De Jongh, A. D., Resick, P. A., Zoellner, L. A., Van Minnen, A., Lee, C. W., Monson, C. M., Foa, E. B., Wheeler, K., ten Broeke, E., Feeny, N., Rauch, S. A. M., Chard, K. M., Mueser, K. T.., Sloan, D. M., van der Gaag, M., Rothbaum, B. O., Neuner, F., de Roos, C., Hehenkamp, L. M. J., Rosner, R., & Bicanic, I. A. (2016). Critical analysis of the current treatment guidelines for complex PTSD in adults. *Depression and Anxiety, 33*(5), 359–369.

Devilly, G. J., Spence, S. H., & Rapee, R. M. (1998). Statistical and reliable change with eye movement desensitization and reprocessing: Treating trauma within a veteran population. *Behavior Therapy, 29*(3), 435–455.

Domhardt, M., & Baumeister, H. (2018). Psychotherapy of adjustment disorders: Current state and future directions. *The World Journal of Biological Psychiatry, 19*(sup1), S21–S35.

Dondanville, K. A., Wachen, J. S., Hale, W. J., Mintz, J., Roache, J. D., Carson, C., Litz, B. T., Yarvis, J. S., Young-McCaughan, S., Peterson, A. L., Resick, P. A., & The STRONG STAR Consortium. (2019). Examination of treatment effects on hazardous drinking among service members with posttraumatic stress disorder. *Journal of Traumatic Stress, 32*(2), 310–316.

Eftekhari, A., Ruzek, J. I., Crowley, J. J., Rosen, C. S., Greenbaum, M. A., & Karlin, B. E. (2013). Effectiveness of national implementation of prolonged exposure therapy in Veterans Affairs care. *JAMA Psychiatry, 70*(9), 949–955.

Ehlers, A., & Clark, D. M. (2000). A cognitive model of posttraumatic stress disorder. *Behaviour Research and Therapy, 38*(4), 319–345.

Ehlers, A., Clark, D. M., Hackmann, A., McManus, F., & Fennell, M. (2005). Cognitive therapy for post-traumatic stress disorder: Development and evaluation. *Behaviour Research and Therapy, 43*(4), 413–431.

Ehlers, A., Clark, D. M., Hackmann, A., McManus, F., Fennell, M., Herbert, C., & Mayou, R. (2003). A randomized controlled trial of cognitive therapy, a self-help booklet, and repeated assessments as early interventions for posttraumatic stress disorder. *Archives of General Psychiatry, 60*(10), 1024–1032.

Ehlers, A., Hackmann, A., Grey, N., Wild, J., Liness, S., Albert, I., Deale, A., Stott, R., & Clark, D. M. (2014). A randomized controlled trial of 7-day intensive and standard weekly cognitive therapy for PTSD and emotion-focused supportive therapy. *American Journal of Psychiatry, 171*, 294–304.

Foa, E. B., Bredemeier, K., Acierno, R., Rosenfield, D., Muzzy, W., Tuerk, P. W., Zandberg, L. J., Hart, S., Young-McCaughan, S., Peterson, A. L., & McLean, C. P. (2022). The efficacy of 90-min versus 60-min sessions of prolonged exposure for PTSD: A randomized controlled trial in active-duty military personnel. *Journal of Consulting and Clinical Pssychology, 90*(6), 503–512.

Foa, E. B., Hembree, E. A., Rothbaum, B. O., & Rausch, S. A. (2019). *Prolonged exposure therapy for PTSD: Emotional processing of traumatic experiences* (2nd ed.), New York: Oxford University Press.

Foa, E. B., McLean, C. P., Zang, Y., Rosenfield, D., Yadin, E., Yarvis, J. S., Mintz, J., Young-McCaughan, S., Borah, E. V., Dondanville, K. A., Fina, B. A., Hall-Clark, B. N., Lichner, T., Litz, B. T., Roache, J., Wright, E. C., Peterson, A. L., & The STRONG

STAR Consortium. (2018). Effect of prolonged exposure therapy delivered over 2 weeks vs 8 weeks vs present-centered therapy on PTSD symptom severity in military personnel: A randomized clinical trial. *JAMA, 319*(4), 354–364.

Forbes, D., Lloyd, D., Nixon, R. D. V., Elliott, P., Varker, T., Perry, D., Bryant, R. A., & Creamer, M. (2012). A multisite randomized controlled effectiveness trial of cognitive processing therapy for military-related posttraumatic stress disorder. *Journal of Anxiety Disorders, 26*(3), 442–452.

Galovski, T. E., Blain, L. M., Mott, J. M., Elwood, L., & Houle, T. (2012). Manualized therapy for PTSD: Flexing the structure of cognitive processing therapy. *Journal of Consulting and Clinical Psychology, 80*(6), 968–981.

Guina, J., Rossetter, S. R., DeRhodes, B. J., Nahhas, R. W., & Welton, R. S. (2015). Benzodiazepines for PTSD: A systematic review and meta-analysis. *Journal of Psychiatric Practice, 21*(4), 281–303.

Harned, M. S., Schmidt, S. C., Korslund, K. E., & Gallop, R. J. (2021). Does adding the Dialectical Behavior Therapy Prolonged Exposure (DBT PE) protocol for PTSD to DBT improve outcomes in public mental health settings? A pilot nonrandomized effectiveness trial with benchmarking. *Behavior Therapy, 52*(3), 639–655.

Held, P., Kovacevic, M., Petrey, K., Meade, E. A., Pridgen, S., Montes, M., Werner, B., Miller, M. L., Smith, D. L., Kaysen, D., & Karnik, N. S. (2022). Treating posttraumatic stress disorder at home in a single week using 1-week virtual massed cognitive processing therapy. *Journal of Traumatic Stress, 35*(4), 1215–1225.

International Society for Traumatic Stress Studies (ISTSS). (2018). ISTSS PTSD prevention and treatment guidelines: Methodology and recommendations. Retrieved from www.istss.org/getattachment/Treating-Trauma/New-ISTSS-Prevention-and-TreatmentGuidelines/ISTSS_PreventionTreatmentGuidelines_FNL.pdf.aspx

Jacoby, V. M., Straud, C. L., Bagley, J. M., Tyler, H., Baker, S. N., Denejkina, A., Sippel, L. M., Kaya, R., Rozek, D. C., Fina, B. A., Dondanville, K. A., & STRONG STAR Training Initiative. (2022). Evidence-based posttraumatic stress disorder treatment in a community sample: Military-affiliated versus civilian patient outcomes. *Journal of Traumatic Stress, 35*(4), 1072–1086.

Jak, A. J., Jurick, S., Crocker, L. D., Sanderson-Cimino, M., Aupperle, R., Rodgers, C. S., Thomas, K. R., Boyd, B., Norman, S. B., Lang, A. J., Keller, A. V., Schiehser, D. M., & Twamley, E. W. (2019). SMART-CPT for veterans with comorbid post-traumatic stress disorder and history of traumatic brain injury: A randomised controlled trial. *Journal of Neurology, Neurosurgery & Psychiatry, 90*(3), 333–341.

Jericho, B., Luo, A., & Berle, D. (2022). Trauma-focused psychotherapies for post-traumatic stress disorder: A systematic review and network meta-analysis. *Acta Psychiatrica Scandinavica, 145*(2), 132–155.

Kaysen, D., Lindgren, K., Zangana, G. A. S., Murray, L., Bass, J., & Bolton, P. (2013). Adaptation of cognitive processing therapy for treatment of torture victims: Experience in Kurdistan, Iraq. *Psychological Trauma: Theory, Research, Practice, and Policy, 5*(2), 184–192.

Lely, J. C., Smid, G. E., Jongedijk, R. A., W. Knipscheer, J., & Kleber, R. J. (2019). The effectiveness of narrative exposure therapy: A review, meta-analysis and meta-regression analysis. *European Journal of Psychotraumatology, 10*(1), 1550344.

LoSavio, S. T., Worley, C. B., Aajmain, S. T., Rosen, C. S., Wiltsey Stirman, S., & Sloan, D. M. (2023). Effectiveness of written exposure therapy for posttraumatic stress disorder in the Department of Veterans Affairs Healthcare System. *Psychological Trauma: Theory, Research, Practice, and Policy, 15,* 748–756.

McDonagh, A., Friedman, M., McHugo, G., Ford, J., Sengupta, A., Mueser, K., Demment, C. C., Fournier, D., Schnurr, P. P., & Descamps, M. (2005). Randomized trial of cognitive-behavioral therapy for chronic posttraumatic stress disorder in adult female survivors of childhood sexual abuse. *Journal of Consulting and Clinical Psychology, 73*(3), 515–524.

McLean, C. P., Foa, E. B., Dondanville, K. A., Haddock, C. K., Miller, M. L., Rauch, S. A., Yarvis, J. S., Wright, E. C., Hall-Clark, B. N., Fina, B. A., Litz, B. T., Mintz, J., Young-McCaughan, S., & Peterson, A. L. (2021). The effects of web-prolonged exposure among military personnel and veterans with posttraumatic stress disorder. *Psychological Trauma: Theory, Research, Practice, and Policy, 13*(6), 621–631.

Morland, L. A., Wells, S. Y., Glassman, L. H., Greene, C. J., Hoffman, J. E., & Rosen, C. S. (2020). Advances in PTSD treatment delivery: Review of findings and clinical considerations for the use of telehealth interventions for PTSD. *Current Treatment Options in Psychiatry, 7,* 221–241.

National Institute for Health and Clinical Practice (NICE). (2018). *Guideline for post-traumatic stress disorder*. London: Author.

Nixon, R. D. (2012). Cognitive processing therapy versus supportive counseling for acute stress disorder following assault: A randomized pilot trial. *Behavior Therapy, 43*(4), 825–836.

Nixon, R. D. V., Best, T., Wilksch, S. R., Angelakis, S., Beatty, L. J., & Weber, N. (2016). Cognitive processing therapy for the treatment of acute stress disorder following sexual assault: A randomised effectiveness study. *Behaviour Change, 33,* 232–250.

O'Donnell, M. L., Metcalf, O., Watson, L., Phelps, A., & Varker, T. (2018). A systematic review of psychological and pharmacological treatments for adjustment disorder in adults. *Journal of Traumatic Stress, 31*(3), 321–331.

Pearson, C. R., Kaysen, D., Huh, D., & Bedard-Gilligan, M. (2019). Randomized control trial of culturally adapted cognitive processing therapy for PTSD substance misuse and HIV sexual risk behavior for Native American women. *AIDS and Behavior, 23,* 695–706.

Pennebaker, J. W., & Beall, S. K. (1986). Confronting a traumatic event: Toward an understanding of inhibition and disease. *Journal of Abnormal Psychology, 95*(3), 274–281.

Peterson, A. L., Mintz, J., Moring, J. C., Straud, C. L., Young-McCaughan, S., McGeary, C. A., McGeary, D. D., Litz, B. T., Velligan, D. I., Macdonald, A., Mata-Galan, E., Holliday, S. L., Dillon, K. H., Roache, J. D., Bira, L. M., Nabity, P. S., Medellin, E. M., Hale, W. J., & Resick, P. A. (2022). In-office, in-home, and telehealth cognitive processing therapy for posttraumatic stress disorder in veterans: A randomized clinical trial. *BMC Psychiatry, 22*(1), 41.

Phoenix Australia Centre for Posttraumatic Mental Health (Phoenix Australia). (2013). *Australian guidelines for the treatment of acute stress disorder and posttraumatic stress disorder*. Melbourne: Author.

Powers, M. B., Halpern, J. M., Ferenschak, M. P., Gillihan, S. J., & Foa, E. B. (2010). A meta-analytic review of prolonged exposure for posttraumatic stress disorder. *Clinical Psychology Review, 30*(6), 635–641.

Renfrey, G., & Spates, C. R. (1994). Eye movement desensitization: A partial dismantling study. *Journal of Behavior Therapy and Experimental Psychiatry, 25*(3), 231–239.

Resick, P. A., Galovski, T. E., Uhlmansiek, M. O. B., Scher, C. D., Clum, G. A., & Young-Xu, Y. (2008). A randomized clinical trial to dismantle components of cognitive processing therapy for posttraumatic stress disorder in female victims of interpersonal violence. *Journal of Consulting and Clinical Psychology, 76*(2), 243–258.

Resick, P. A., Monson, C. M., & Chard, K. M. (2024). *Cognitive processing therapy for PTSD: A comprehensive therapist manual* (2nd ed.). New York: Guilford.

Resick, P. A., Nishith, P., Weaver, T. L., Astin, M. C., & Feuer, C. A. (2002). A comparison of cognitive-processing therapy with prolonged exposure and a waiting condition for the treatment of chronic posttraumatic stress disorder in female rape victims. *Journal of Consulting and Clinical Psychology, 70*(4), 867–879.

Resick, P. A., & Schnicke, M. K. (1993). *Cognitive processing therapy for rape victims: A treatment manual.* Newbury Park, CA: Sage Publications.

Resick, P. A., Wachen, J. S., Dondanville, K. A., LoSavio, S. T., Young-McCaughan, S., Yarvis, J. S., Pruiksma, K. E., Blankenship, A., Jacoby, V., Peterson, A. L., Mintz, J., & Strong Star Consortium. (2021). Variable-length cognitive processing therapy for post-traumatic stress disorder in active duty military: Outcomes and predictors. *Behaviour Research and Therapy, 141*, 103846.

Resick, P. A., Wachen, J. S., Mintz, J., Young-McCaughan, S., Roache, J. D., Borah, A. M., Borah, E. V., Dondanville, K. A., Hembree, E. A., Litz, B. T., & Peterson, A. L. (2015). A randomized clinical trial of group cognitive processing therapy compared with group present-centered therapy for PTSD among active duty military personnel. *Journal of Consulting and Clinical Osychology, 83*(6), 1058–1068.

Robjant, K., & Fazel, M. (2010). The emerging evidence for narrative exposure therapy: A review. *Clinical Psychology Review, 30*(8), 1030–1039.

Schauer, M., Neuner, F., & Elbert, T. (2011). *Narrative exposure therapy: A short-term treatment for traumatic stress disorders* (2nd ed.). Hogrefe Publishing.

Schnurr, P. P., Chard, K. M., Ruzek, J. I., Chow, B. K., Resick, P. A., Foa, E. B., Marx, B. P., Friedman, M. J., Bovin, M. J., Caudle, K. L., Castillo, D., Curry, K. T., Hollifield, M., Huang, G. D., Chee, C. L., Astin, M. C., Dickstein, B., Renner, K., Clancy, C. P., Collie, C., Maieritsch, K., Bailey, S., Thompson, K., Messina, M., Franklin, L., Lindley, S., Kattar, K., Luedtke, B., Romesser, J., McQuaid, J., Sylvers, P., Varkovitzky, R., Davis, L., MacVicar, D., & Shih, M. C. (2022). Comparison of prolonged exposure vs cognitive processing therapy for treatment of posttraumatic stress disorder among US veterans: A randomized clinical trial. *JAMA Network Open, 5*(1), e2136921–e2136921.

Schnurr, P. P., Friedman, M. J., Engel, C. C., Foa, E. B., Shea, M. T., Chow, B. K., Resick, P. A., Thurston, V., Orsillo, S. M., Haug, R., Turner, C., & Bernardy, N. (2007). Cognitive behavioral therapy for posttraumatic stress disorder in women: A randomized controlled trial. *JAMA, 297*(8), 820–830.

Schnurr, P. P., Friedman, M. J., Foy, D. W., Shea, M. T., Hsieh, F. Y., Lavori, P. W., Glynn, S. M., Wattenberg, M., & & Bernardy, N. C. (2003). Randomized trial of trauma-focused group therapy for posttraumatic stress disorder: Results from a Department of Veterans Affairs cooperative study. *Archives of General Psychiatry, 60*(5), 481–489.

Shapiro, F. (1989). Eye movement desensitization: A new treatment for post-traumatic stress disorder. *Journal of Behavior Therapy and Experimental Psychiatry, 20*(3), 211–217.

Shapiro, F. (2018). *Eye movement desensitization and reprocessing: Basic principles, protocols, and procedures* (3rd ed.). New York: Guilford Press.

Shear, M. K. (2015). Complicated grief treatment (CGT) for prolonged grief disorder. In U. Schnyder & M. Cloitre (Eds.) *Evidence based treatments for trauma-related psychological disorders: A practical guide for clinicians* (pp. 299–314). Cham: Springer International Publishing.

Sloan, D. M., Lee, D. J., Litwack, S. D., Sawyer, A. T., & Marx, B. P. (2013). Written exposure therapy for veterans diagnosed with PTSD: A pilot study. *Journal of Traumatic Stress, 26*(6), 776–779.

Sloan, D. M., & Marx, B. P. (2019). *Written exposure therapy for PTSD: A brief treatment approach for mental health professionals.* Washington, D.C.: American Psychological Association.

Sloan, D. M., Marx, B. P., Acierno, R., Messina, M., Muzzy, W., Gallagher, M. W., Littwack, S., & Sloan, C. (2023). Written Exposure Therapy vs Prolonged Exposure Therapy in the treatment of posttraumatic stress disorder: A randomized clinical trial. *JAMA Psychiatry, 80*(11), 1093–1100. Advance online publication.

Sloan, D. M., Marx, B. P., Bovin, M. J., Feinstein, B. A., & Gallagher, M. W. (2012). Written exposure as an intervention for PTSD: A randomized clinical trial with motor vehicle accident survivors. *Behaviour Research and Therapy, 50*(10), 627–635.

Sloan, D. M., Marx, B. P., Lee, D. J., & Resick, P. A. (2018). A brief exposure-based treatment vs cognitive processing therapy for posttraumatic stress disorder: A randomized noninferiority clinical trial. *JAMA Psychiatry, 75*(3), 233–239.

Sloan, D. M., Marx, B. P., Resick, P. A., Young-McCaughan, S., Dondanville, K. A., Straud, C. L., Mintz, J., Litz, B. T., Peterson, A. L., & The STRONG STAR Consortium. (2022). Effect of written exposure therapy vs cognitive processing therapy on increasing treatment efficiency among military service members with posttraumatic stress disorder: A randomized noninferiority trial. *JAMA Network Open, 5*(1), e2140911–e2140911.

Sloan, D. M., Sawyer, A. T., Lowmaster, S. E., Wernick, J., & Marx, B. P. (2015). Efficacy of narrative writing as an intervention for PTSD: Does the evidence support its use? *Journal of Contemporary Psychotherapy, 45*, 215–225.

Sripada, R. K., & Rauch, S. A. (2015). Between-session and within-session habituation in prolonged exposure therapy for posttraumatic stress disorder: A hierarchical linear modeling approach. *Journal of Anxiety Disorders, 30*, 81–87.

Surís, A., Link-Malcolm, J., Chard, K., Ahn, C., & North, C. (2013). A randomized clinical trial of cognitive processing therapy for veterans with PTSD related to military sexual trauma. *Journal of Traumatic Stress, 26*(1), 28–37.

Szuhany, K. L., Malgaroli, M., Miron, C. D., & Simon, N. M. (2021). Prolonged grief disorder: Course, diagnosis, assessment, and treatment. *Focus, 19*(2), 161–172.

Takagishi, Y., Ito, M., Kanie, A., Morita, N., Makino, M., Katayanagi, A., Sato, T., Imamura, F., Nakajima, S., Oe, Y., Kashimura, M., Kikuchi, A., Narisawa, T., & Horikoshi, M. (2023). Feasibility, acceptability, and preliminary efficacy of cognitive processing therapy in Japanese patients with posttraumatic stress disorder. *Journal of Traumatic Stress, 36*(1), 205–217.

Taylor, D. J., Pruiksma, K. E., Mintz, J., Slavish, D. C., Wardle-Pinkston, S., Dietch, J. R., Dondanville, K. A., Young-McCaughan, S., Nicholson, K. L., Litz, B. T., Keane, T. M., Peteson, A. L., Resick, P. A., & the Consortium to Alleviate PTSD. (2023). Treatment of comorbid sleep disorders and posttraumatic stress disorder in US active duty military personnel: A pilot randomized clinical trial. *Journal of Traumatic Stress, 36*, 712–726.

Thompson-Hollands, J., Marx, B. P., Lee, D. J., Resick, P. A., & Sloan, D. M. (2018). Long-term treatment gains of a brief exposure-based treatment for PTSD. *Depression and Anxiety, 35*, 985–991.

U.S. Department of Veterans Affairs and Department of Defense (VA/DoD) (2023). VA/DoD clinical practice guideline for the management of posttraumatic stress disorder and acute stress disorder. Retrieved from https://www.healthquality.va.gov/guidelines/MH/ptsd/VA-DoD-CPG-PTSD-Full-CPG.pdf

van Minnen, A., & Foa, E. B. (2006). The effect of imaginal exposure length on outcome of treatment for PTSD. *Journal of Traumatic Stress: Official Publication of the International Society for Traumatic Stress Studies, 19*(4), 427–438.

Watts, B. V., Schnurr, P. P., Mayo, L., Young-Xu, Y., Weeks, W. B., & Friedman, M. J. (2013). Meta-analysis of the efficacy of treatments for posttraumatic stress disorder. *The Journal of Clinical Psychiatry, 74*(6), 11710.

Wells, S. Y., LoSavio, S. T., Patel, T. A., Evans, M. K., Beckham, J. C., Calhoun, P., & Dedert, E. A. (2022). Contingency management and cognitive behavior therapy for smoking cessation among veterans with posttraumatic stress disorder: Design and methodology of a randomized clinical trial. *Contemporary Clinical Trials, 119*, 106839.

Wittouck, C., Van Autreve, S., De Jaegere, E., Portzky, G., & van Heeringen, K. (2011). The prevention and treatment of complicated grief: A meta-analysis. *Clinical Psychology Review, 31*(1), 69–78.

7

Dissemination of Treatment: From Research to Practice

Over the last few decades, researchers have produced volumes of literature on the most effective treatments for posttraumatic stress disorder (PTSD); however, treatment development and refinement has substantially outpaced dissemination and implementation of evidence-based treatments into patient care settings. Despite several treatment options with strong evidence supporting their use (see Chapter 6), the reach of evidence-based treatments has continued to be limited by a "research-practice gap". Significant efforts have been made over the last 20 years to bring PTSD treatments into the settings where patients receive care, but there is still a long way to go to ensure that the recommended interventions most likely to result in improvement are available on the front lines of mental health care.

Data from the National Epidemiologic Survey on Alcohol and Related Conditions-III indicated that 24% of those with lifetime PTSD and 30% of those with past-year PTSD accessed PTSD treatment within the last year (Hale et al., 2018). However, few of those seeking treatment for PTSD will receive one of the evidence-based treatments discussed in Chapter 6. An entire field of "implementation science" has developed to address these issues, focused on the study of methods that facilitate uptake of evidence-based strategies into routine practice (e.g., see Bauer & Kirchner, 2020). Researchers in this field aim to identify and deploy effective implementation strategies that capitalize on facilitators and address barriers to widespread use of evidence-based practices.

Of course, implementation challenges are not unique to PTSD treatments. However, trauma-focused treatments face significant challenges in their dissemination

DOI: 10.4324/9780429317934-7

because the most effective treatment strategies typically involve approaching trauma memories, which can seem daunting for both patients and clinicians. In this chapter, we will review PTSD treatment dissemination and implementation efforts, including their successes and challenges, and then we will provide an overview of some of the ongoing barriers to implementing and sustaining evidence-based PTSD treatments in patient care settings that must be overcome in future years to increase the reach of evidence-based PTSD treatments.

Dissemination and Implementation Programs

The most effective and well-studied treatments for PTSD that we have today, cognitive processing therapy (CPT) and prolonged exposure (PE), emerged in the 1980s. Efforts have been ongoing since that time to optimize the delivery of these treatments and then to disseminate them to mental healthcare settings, with the most significant dissemination efforts initially taking off in the early 2000s. Below we describe some of these training initiatives in the United States, including in the Department of Veterans Affairs (VA) and community, as well as worldwide.

Dissemination Efforts in the US Department of Veterans Affairs

One healthcare system that has been a leader in dissemination and implementation of evidence-based treatments for trauma-related disorders is the US Veterans Health Administration (VHA), which is the healthcare delivery arm of the VA. VHA is the largest healthcare system in the United States and, owing to the large proportion of veterans suffering from PTSD due to both military and civilian traumas, VHA has invested substantially in PTSD treatment development, refinement, training, and delivery. Beginning in 2007, VHA began to "roll out" evidence-based PTSD treatments including CPT and PE (Chard et al., 2012; Eftekhari et al., 2013; Karlin et al., 2010).

To date, thousands of mental health providers have been formally trained to deliver CPT and/or PE. (Significantly more providers—over 11,000—have been trained in CPT). VA policy also mandates that patients with PTSD have access to these first-line treatments. VHA has continued to train providers in CPT and PE each year. Providers are also now being trained throughout VHA in written exposure therapy (WET; Worley et al., 2023).

VHA has set a standard for competency-based training for PTSD treatments, which typically includes both a workshop—involving didactic and experiential components such as role play, video demonstrations, and discussion of cases examples—and clinical case consultation—weekly phone or video calls, led by a treatment expert, during which clinicians get assistance applying the model to their training cases. Clinicians are typically required to competently deliver the treatment model to two patient cases under the guidance of a consultant as part of training. Clinicians also share patient symptom outcomes, as well as work samples as part of this process. For example, for PE training in VHA, clinicians submit audio recordings of their sessions. For WET, clinicians read their patients' trauma narratives aloud in consultation. For CPT, clinicians share patient materials such as impact statements, stuck point logs, trauma accounts, and/or worksheets. Consultation helps clinicians learn how to skillfully apply the treatment protocol to their cases, balancing fidelity to the protocol with flexibility to the individual case presentation. Such post-workshop clinical case consultation has been shown to improve patient outcomes for trauma-focused treatments (Charney et al., 2019; Foa et al., 2020), especially when therapists have lower initial self-efficacy (Pace et al., 2021). Thus, consultation may build both mastery in the therapy and confidence applying it to cases.

Successes and Challenges

Across PTSD treatment models, program evaluation data show that patients treated by VHA providers obtain good treatment outcomes, including VHA providers delivering their initial training cases while in consultation (Chard et al., 2012; Eftekhari et al., 2013; LoSavio et al., 2023). These findings are promising and suggest that professional therapists can develop sufficient mastery in these models and obtain good clinical outcomes, even with veteran patients, who sometimes present with more clinical complexity.

Unfortunately, despite these notable dissemination efforts, the reach of evidence-based protocols has remained less than optimal, even in this healthcare system valuing evidence-based practices. Despite VHA's strong commitment to training, a review of national VHA evidence-based psychotherapy trends showed low rates of treatment delivery: The highest annual rates of CPT and PE delivery over the period of 2001–2014 were 15% and 5%, respectively, with even lower rates of minimally adequate doses of treatment (eight or more sessions, 1–5%; Maguen et al., 2020). These and other collateral data suggest that even providers trained in CPT and PE—in healthcare settings required to offer them—do not necessarily consistently deliver evidence-based treatments.

Another issue is that even when providers and programs report using evidence-based protocols, they sometimes deliver them without strict adherence to the essential elements of the protocols, which may dampen treatment effectiveness. One study indicated that in outpatient PTSD clinics in VHA, only 52% of CPT providers "very often" adhered to the CPT manual (Finley et al., 2015). Lower treatment fidelity may contribute to some recent observations of less impressive outcomes in VHA routine care than typically seen in clinical trials (Maguen et al., 2023).

Some of the underutilization observed in VHA has been associated with characteristics of the specific clinics in which treatments are being delivered. For example, clinics with higher reach of evidence-based treatments are more likely to have staff members who describe a clinic mission to provide evidence-based treatments, leadership championing evidence-based practices, and positive beliefs about the interventions (Sayer et al., 2017).

Taken together, efforts to disseminate first-line PTSD treatments in VHA highlight the value of system-wide training and organizational support for training. However, that reach of evidence-based treatments and fidelity to the protocol remain suboptimal—even in a healthcare system committed to evidence-based practices and with evidence-based care mandates—suggests that additional steps may be needed to optimize dissemination and implementation of best practices for PTSD. Building on some community training efforts described in the next session, some VHA training programs are now including additional training elements, such as implementation support, to help facilitate sustainability long-term (Worley et al., 2023).

US Community-Based Dissemination Efforts

In the community, a number of training initiatives have been launched to spread evidence-based PTSD treatments to patients seeking care outside of VHA. Community-based initiatives offer training, sometimes subsidized to increase access, to a wide range of mental health providers operating out of hospitals, mental health organizations, or private practice settings. Training in the community is extremely variable: Clinicians vary widely in their work setting and training background, and a wide range of training programs have been deployed, differing in their training approaches and outcomes reported (if reported at all).

Clinicians in the community may attempt to deliver an evidence-based treatment without formal training, such as after reading the treatment manual or while receiving supervision before being licensed. Several organizations offer treatment workshops for evidence-based PTSD treatments, so clinicians may also attend a treatment workshop. However, as noted above, research has shown the value of clinical case consultation, particularly for evidence-based PTSD treatments. Some community-based training programs offer both workshop and consultation, as is typically done in VHA (e.g., Dondanville et al., 2021). Fewer programs have also provided implementation support to facilitate integration of the evidence-based treatment into the practice setting and foster sustainability after training has ended (LoSavio, Dillon, Murphy, Goetz, et al., 2019). These enhanced training models—sometimes called Learning Communities or Learning Collaboratives—may further improve implementation outcomes.

Learning Collaboratives involve additional components that go beyond the workshop plus consultation model and incorporate additional clinical training and implementation support elements. In addition to the training components part of workshop plus consultation models, Learning Collaboratives can also include (1) team-based training, where multiple clinicians from the same organization participate; (2) involvement of a "senior leader", who is someone with administrative authority within the organization who can help support implementation of the intervention; (3) multiple, face-to-face learning sessions separated by supported action periods; (4) evaluation of work samples, such as fidelity rating of recorded sessions; (5) expert guidance from an implementation specialist who helps the team build organizational capacity and implement the treatment into their specific setting; (6) monitoring of "monthly metrics" to assess how well the intervention is implemented into the service setting; (7) cross-site sharing of challenges, successes, products, and processes; and (8) an emphasis on fostering sustainability of the treatment, such as developing procedures to monitor and support the intervention after training (Nadeem et al., 2013). There are data to suggest that those trained in a Learning Collaborative model versus a less intensive training model ultimately serve more patients (Brown et al., 2014). Thus, the additional training elements may overcome some of the shortcomings of other training programs and enhance implementation outcomes.

Some teams operating community-based training programs have published their program evaluation data, demonstrating excellent patient outcomes with clinicians delivering the PTSD treatment models to their first training cases. Community-based training programs also have shown success targeting clinician- and organization-level outcomes such as sustainability of the intervention. In one example of the Learning Collaborative training approach, researchers trained teams of community clinicians in CPT over the course of a year. Six months after training, 95% of rostered clinicians had continued to deliver CPT, and 100% of the agencies continued to offer CPT (LoSavio, Dillon, Murphy, Goetz, et al., 2019).

Some teams have used models that incorporate some but not all of the elements of a Learning Collaborative, such as a "Learning Community" framework that builds upon the workshop-plus-consultation model. For example, the STRONG STAR Training Initiative offers training in CPT, PE, WET, and other evidence-based models and provides, in addition to the workshop and consultation, web-based pre-workshop training in assessment of PTSD, post-workshop advanced training webinars, and an online provider portal with access to treatment delivery resources including therapy demonstration videos and patient symptom monitoring tools, plus the availability of organizational consultation (Dondanville et al., 2021). Clinicians trained in these Learning Communities have evidenced high rates of continuing to deliver CPT and PE at 6 and 12 months post-training: 95% and 87% for CPT at 6 and 12 months, respectively, and 72% and 77% for PE at 6 and 12 months, respectively (Dondanville et al., 2022).

Dissemination Efforts Across the World

As noted in Chapter 6, clinical practice guidelines consistently recommend trauma-focused cognitive behavioral therapies for the treatment of PTSD. This includes the guidelines from the International Society for Traumatic Stress Studies (ISTSS, 2018), the National Institute for Health and Care Excellence (NICE, 2018), and the Phoenix Australia Centre for Posttraumatic Mental Health (Phoenix Australia, 2013). Evidence-based PTSD treatments have been delivered outside the United States, in countries such as Australia, Cambodia, Canada, Germany, Japan, Korea, Iraq, and the Democratic Republic of Congo (Bass et al., 2013; Clemans et al., 2021; Forbes et al., 2012; Kaysen et al., 2013; Monson et al., 2018; Park et al., 2021; Rosner et al., 2019; Takagishi et al., 2023). However, formal implementation programs to disseminate these treatments widely have been scarcer.

One notable implementation example involves CPT training that was launched in 2012 across a national community-based veterans mental health service in Australia. Training elements include consultation, leadership support, and integration of PTSD-specific screening and symptom monitoring tools. The implementation program has shown large effect sizes for patients' PTSD symptoms, as well as good clinician treatment fidelity (Lloyd et al., 2015). This program is promising for being a national implementation program and having outcomes in routine care settings that were on par with those typically observed in clinical trials.

The Canadian Institute for Research also funded an implementation program in Canada with the agreement that the program would also be a research project (Monson et al., 2018). As part of the research, the authors studied different formats of case consultation, not just to measure therapist fidelity but also to study patient outcomes. Therapists across Canada were trained in CPT and then randomly assigned to one of three conditions: No consultation (but delayed feedback on fidelity at the end of the study), standard consultation that included weekly group online discussion of cases, and consultation including audio review of segments of therapy. The consultation groups lasted for six months. Although they predicted that listening to clips from therapy would be superior, in fact, the standard discussion of cases proved to have better outcomes for patients. They concluded that listening to an audio clip of a specific patient was not as beneficial as having everyone discuss their progress and problems with all their patients.

In the United Kingdom, the Improving Access to Psychological Therapies (IAPT) program was launched to make evidence-based psychological treatments recommended by NICE guidelines (broadly, not just PTSD) widely available within the National Health Service (Clark, 2018). This has included training of providers in cognitive behavioral therapies (e.g., PE) and eye movement desensitization and reprocessing (EMDR) for PTSD. Researchers in the United Kingdom have also explored ways of providing treatment when patients cannot access therapists. Ehlers et al. (2023) compared two therapist-assisted internet-based treatments for PTSD to a three-month waitlist with usual National Health Service care (general practitioner and/or medications). The two internet conditions were iCT-PTSD (internet cognitive therapy for PTSD) or iStress-PTSD (stress management program to learn and practice coping skills). The two internet treatments were augmented with 20-minute weekly phone calls during treatment and three monthly phone calls in the booster phase. Both internet therapies were superior to the waitlist, but iCT-PTSD was superior to iStress-PTSD. The therapies had similar outcomes to in-person therapy with half the therapist time.

In low- and middle-income countries, there is an even greater discrepancy between traumatic stress and access to evidence-based treatment, with estimates suggesting that as many as 90% of those needing services do not receive any treatment (Murray et al., 2014). Implementation efforts have been undertaken to address international crises including disasters and geopolitical conflict. Studying dissemination and implementation in conflict-affected settings, Murray and colleagues (2014) have highlighted challenges and successes of efforts to increase the availability of effective interventions, such as the training of lay or nonspecialist providers to address shortages of local mental health professionals; working closely with local organizations and developing flexible implementation plans including options for remote treatment and supervision to ensure safety; delivering care in community centers or religious spaces; using non-stigmatizing language; and engaging local leaders to increase acceptability and feasibility of care.

Successes and Challenges

Again, excellent training outcomes are a frequent outcome of community-based training programs. The addition of implementation supports may further strengthen key outcomes including fidelity, reach, and sustainability post-training.

Although good estimates are hard to come by, use of evidence-based PTSD treatments is almost certainly lower in the community than in VHA. The average patient presenting for PTSD treatment in the community is unlikely to receive one of the evidence-based treatments discussed in this book (McHugh & Barlow, 2010). Awareness of and access to training are key limiting factors, with many busy clinicians unaware of or disincentivized to pursue training, which can be time-consuming and costly. The greater availability of live, remote training in recent years may partially mitigate expenses associated with traveling for training, but the overall reach of training remains a challenge.

Funding for training is also inconsistent, and research suggests that state-level investment in evidence-based treatments has declined, not increased over time (Bruns et al., 2015). Overall, the need for training in evidence-based treatment far exceeds the availability of affordable training.

Additionally, when mandates for evidence-based treatment delivery are not in place, and there are not other internal or external pressures to deliver evidence-based treatments, such as from managed care organizations, it falls upon motivated clinicians and organizations to pursue training. As discussed further later in this chapter, a range of factors may limit such efforts.

Common Implementation Challenges

Barriers to the widespread availability of evidence-based PTSD treatment exist at numerous levels, including the policy, organizational, clinic, provider, patient, and intervention levels (Damschroder et al., 2009; Karlin & Cross, 2014). At the policy level, factors such as funding for training and reimbursement for services can inform which treatments are trained in and delivered. Although there are some state-funded training initiatives, more commonly for child than adult treatments, many initiatives to train community providers in evidence-based treatments are foundation-funded (e.g., Dondanville et al., 2021; LoSavio, Dillon, Murphy, Goetz, et al., 2019). Thus, due to lack of continuous funding streams, community-based training is often limited, especially at subsidized rates that might be attainable for community providers, and sometimes limited to providers servicing certain patient populations.

Within organizations, factors such as implementation leadership, organizational readiness to implement the intervention, and implementation climate influence how well new interventions are integrated and sustained, as do more pragmatic factors like staffing and availability of resources. Qualitative research in VHA has differentiated clinics with high versus low levels of evidence-based treatment reach based on factors such as lack of dedicated time and resources, strong implementation leadership, and a supportive peer network (Cook, Dinnen, et al., 2015; Sayer et al., 2017).

Provider-level factors also affect which treatments will be offered and delivered to patients. Lack of knowledge about treatments, low provider skill or self-efficacy to deliver a specific treatment, and provider negative attitudes toward an evidence-based treatment might limit treatment reach (Cook et al., 2014). Because of how common provider concerns about trauma-focused treatments are, we discuss these in greater detail later.

Related to provider-level beliefs and attitudes are characteristics of the intervention itself, including the evidence for the intervention and its perceived advantage over other interventions, adaptability, complexity, and costs (Damschroder et al., 2009). Interventions that are perceived as not only effective but also easy to learn, easy to try out, well packaged, and adaptable to fit the setting are more likely to be implemented (Cook, Thompson, & Schnurr, 2015). Typically, the people developing and studying interventions are not necessarily the same individuals—or even at the same institutions—as those who most commonly deliver them. Thus, treatments may not be acceptable or appealing to end users.

Finally, patients also have a role in selecting interventions that influence the ultimate adoption of evidence-based treatments. Even if organizations and clinicians offer evidence-based treatments, patients must opt into them. Whereas drug companies offer direct marketing to consumers, patients seeking psychotherapy are rarely aware of the range of treatment options, or their comparative effectiveness (Kehle-Forbes et al., 2022). Patients also may have doubts and concerns about particular treatment approaches that may lead them to select more appealing but potentially less effective interventions. For example, patients may prefer treatments that focus on coping with disabling PTSD symptoms rather than interventions that resolve them. Strategies such as patient education about treatment options during clinic orientation and shared decision-making processes can help keep patients informed about treatment options and engage them in the treatment selection process (Schumm et al., 2015).

Perceptions of Trauma-Focused Treatments

While clinician attitudes and beliefs about interventions are relevant across disorders, and indeed, clinicians have concerns about evidence-based treatments and manualized treatments broadly (Addis et al., 1999; DiMeo et al., 2012), treatments for PTSD in particular pose specific challenges. One issue is that the most effective and well-studied interventions for PTSD are trauma-focused treatments, or treatments that focus on (and typically involve talking and/or writing about) the traumatic event directly. While focusing on day-to-day stressors works well for some disorders like depression and generalized anxiety disorder, trauma-related disorders are unique in that many of the everyday problems people experience stem from the traumatic event itself, including the meaning that they made of it and their avoidance of its memory. However, many patients are reluctant to talk or think about their traumatic event because of the distress it can evoke. This can be conceptualized as avoidance, a key symptom of PTSD (American Psychiatric Association, 2022). In response to this avoidance, many well-intentioned providers observe this reluctance or distress and decide not to press their client about discussing the trauma. Therefore, in an effort to not upset their patients, many providers refrain from delivering trauma-focused treatments altogether, or they may pick and choose which elements of a treatment to include, leaving out key elements that are central to the effectiveness of the treatment. These provider behaviors may ultimately prevent patients from receiving the most evidence-based approaches. Contrary to these concerns, although patients sometimes experience distress when they stop avoiding and start processing the trauma, research shows that such distress tends to be temporary, followed by symptom reduction (e.g., Larsen et al., 2022; see LoSavio et al. (2024) and van Minnen et al. (2012) for evidence pertaining to many common therapist concerns). Some evidence-based PTSD treatments also involve exposure (e.g., PE, WET), and it is well documented that many therapists have doubts and concerns about delivering exposure-based interventions (e.g., van Minnen et al., 2012). Perhaps most commonly, clinicians express concern that conducting exposure will destabilize patients and exacerbate PTSD and other comorbid symptoms. Even for treatments that do not involve exposure and focus on cognitive strategies, clinicians still report concerns about making clients worse by discussing the trauma, as well as concerns that treatment will be insufficient to address the range of problems their "complex" clients face (LoSavio, Dillon, Murphy, & Resick, 2019; LoSavio et al., 2024).

While clinician concerns about trauma-focused treatments abound, it is promising to note that even if providers have concerns about trauma-focused treatments initially, these tend to decrease if they participate in training and see training cases in consultation (LoSavio, Dillon, Murphy, Resick et al., 2019; Ruzek et al., 2016). Thus, addressing common therapist concerns is an important aspect to increasing participation in training and the reach of evidence-based treatments.

Treatment Fidelity

An additional issue is that even providers who attend training do not necessarily continue to implement the interventions with fidelity. This "therapist drift" is problematic because fidelity is linked to treatment effectiveness (Farmer et al., 2017; Holder et al., 2018; Marques et al., 2019; Stirman et al., 2021).

A substantial portion of clinicians omit core elements of evidence-based treatments when delivering them after training and in routine care (Finley et al., 2015; Marques et al., 2019; Thompson et al., 2018; Wilk et al., 2013). For example, in a study of Army behavioral health providers, only 15% of providers reported using all of the elements of CPT (Wilk et al., 2013). Interestingly, frequency of evidence-based treatment use appears to be associated with treatment fidelity. One study of VA residential treatment providers found that frequent CPT users delivered key components of CPT fairly consistently, whereas occasional and rare CPT users (<50% of clients) delivered key components less often (Thompson et al., 2018).

Delivery of core elements is, in some cases, linked to provider concerns about treatment. For example, having more negative beliefs about exposure is associated with more cautious delivery of interventions, such as creating a less ambitious exposure hierarchy, choosing less anxiety-provoking items, and greater attempts to minimize patient anxiety, including incorporating relaxation strategies not part of the protocol (Deacon et al., 2013; Farrell et al., 2013). These findings highlight the importance of consultation so that clinicians can get support on their cases and discuss their concerns with a knowledgeable treatment provider.

While adherence to the core elements of a treatment—its active ingredients—is essential to retain the effectiveness of treatments when they leave research settings, adaptations have also been made and tested when delivering evidence-based treatments in novel contexts. Some researchers have dubbed modifications as "fidelity-consistent" if they are minor and do not significantly change the treatment or "fidelity-inconsistent" if they meaningfully change the protocol (Marques et al., 2019). Research suggests that minor tweaks to the protocol, such as using more culturally relevant examples or using different terms for concepts, can have positive effects on the treatment outcome (Marques et al., 2019). Other changes to protocols that appear to improve or not affect outcomes include altering the number of sessions and delivering sessions more closely together (Galovski et al., 2012; Wachen et al., 2019). However, leaving out key treatment elements is associated with worse outcomes. Thus, fidelity is an important implementation outcome worthy of attention during and after training.

Summary and Future Directions

Despite substantial efforts to disseminate first-line PTSD treatments, continued work is needed to narrow the gap between research and practice and ensure that those struggling with trauma and PTSD receive the most effective care. Policies that promote evidence-based care, organizational support, and competency-based training programs have contributed to the spread of evidence-based PTSD treatments and allowed for thousands of mental health providers to be trained in these models and countless patients to receive high-quality care. Nonetheless, uptake of evidence-based PTSD treatments remains low, especially in the community, but even in settings that have prioritized training like VHA. Thus, greater efforts are needed to turn the tide and make evidence-based treatments the primary approaches available on the front lines of mental healthcare.

A shift from primarily in-person to more remote-based training has opened opportunities for more clinicians to participate in training. However, additional barriers, such as therapist attitudes about trauma-focused treatments, continue to threaten the spread of best practices. Multipronged approaches addressing policy-, organization-, clinician-, and patient-level barriers are needed to advance implementation.

More and more, researchers are being encouraged to include stakeholders in their research programs to ensure that treatments are not only effective but also meet the needs of eventual end users including clinicians and patients. Particularly in the United States, managed care is likely to play a part in the successful implementation of evidence-based treatments, given their role in setting reimbursement rates and influencing what services are offered and can be billed. Emphasizing evidence-based treatments in mental health training programs would also increase the reach of such treatments. Ongoing research in the area of implementation science continues to inform the field about what strategies for training work best and under what conditions (Powell et al., 2017). Future efforts may help further determine optimal training and implementation strategies for various providers, treatments, and service settings to ensure that individuals affected by traumatic stress have access to effective care.

References

Addis, M. E., Wade, W. A., & Hatgis, C. (1999). Barriers to dissemination of evidence-based practices: Addressing practitioners' concerns about manual-based psychotherapies. *Clinical Psychology: Science and Practice, 6*(4), 430–441.

American Psychiatric Association. (2022). *Diagnostic and statistical manual of mental disorders* (5th ed., text rev.). Washington D.C.: American Psychiatric Association.

Bass, J. K., Annan, J., McIvor Murray, S., Kaysen, D., Griffiths, S., Cetinoglu, T., Wachter, K., Murray, L. K., & Bolton, P. A. (2013). Controlled trial of psychotherapy for Congolese survivors of sexual violence. *New England Journal of Medicine, 368*(23), 2182–2191.

Bauer, M. S., & Kirchner, J. (2020). Implementation science: What is it and why should I care? *Psychiatry Research, 283*, 112376.

Brown, C. H., Chamberlain, P., Saldana, L., Padgett, C., Wang, W., & Cruden, G. (2014). Evaluation of two implementation strategies in 51 child county public service systems in two states: Results of a cluster randomized head-to-head implementation trial. *Implementation Science, 9*(1), 1–15.

Bruns, E. J., Pullmann, M. D., Kerns, S. E., Hensley, S., Lutterman, T., & Hoagwood, K. E. (2015). How research-based is our policy-making? Implementation of evidence-based treatments by state behavioral health systems, 2001–2012. *Implementation Science, 10*(1), A40.

Chard, K. M., Ricksecker, E. G., Healy, E. T., Karlin, B. E., & Resick, P. A. (2012). Dissemination and experience with cognitive processing therapy. *Journal of Rehabilitation Research & Development, 49*(5), 667–678.

Charney, M. E., Chow, L., Jakubovic, R. J., Federico, L. E., Goetter, E. M., Baier, A. L.,…, & Simon, N. M. (2019). Training community providers in evidence-based treatment for PTSD: Outcomes of a novel consultation program. *Psychological Trauma: Theory, Research, Practice, and Policy, 11*(7), 793–801.

Clark, D. M. (2018). Realizing the mass public benefit of evidence-based psychological therapies: The IAPT program. *Annual Review of Clinical Psychology, 14*, 159–183.

Clemans, T.A., White, K.L., Fuessel-Hermann, D., Bryan, C.J., and Resick, P.A. (2021). Acceptability, feasibility, and preliminary effectiveness of group cognitive processing therapy with female adolescent survivors of commercial sexual exploitation in Cambodia. *Journal of Child and Adolescent Trauma, 14*, 571–583.

Cook, J. M., Dinnen, S., Simiola, V., Thompson, R., & Schnurr, P. P. (2014). VA residential provider perceptions of dissuading factors to the use of two evidence-based PTSD treatments. *Professional Psychology: Research and Practice, 45*(2), 136–142.

Cook, J. M., Dinnen, S., Thompson, R., Ruzek, J., Coyne, J. C., & Schnurr, P. P. (2015). A quantitative test of an implementation framework in 38 VA residential PTSD programs. *Administration and Policy in Mental Health and Mental Health Services Research, 42,* 462–473.

Cook, J. M., Thompson, R., & Schnurr, P. P. (2015). Perceived characteristics of intervention scale: Development and psychometric properties. *Assessment, 22*(6), 704–714.

Damschroder, L. J., Aron, D. C., Keith, R. E., Kirsh, S. R., Alexander, J. A., & Lowery, J. C. (2009). Fostering implementation of health services research findings into practice: A consolidated framework for advancing implementation science. *Implementation Science, 4*(1), 1–15.

Deacon, B. J., Farrell, N. R., Kemp, J. J., Dixon, L. J., Sy, J. T., Zhang, A. R., & McGrath, P. B. (2013). Assessing therapist reservations about exposure therapy for anxiety disorders: The Therapist Beliefs about Exposure Scale. *Journal of Anxiety Disorders, 27*(8), 772–780.

DiMeo, M. A., Moore, G. K., & Lichtenstein, C. (2012). Relationship of evidence-based practice and treatments: A survey of community mental health providers. *Journal of Community Psychology, 40*(3), 341–357.

Dondanville, K. A., Fina, B. A., Straud, C. L., Finley, E. P., Tyler, H., Jacoby, V., Blount, T. H., Moring, J. C., Pruiksma, K. E., Blankenship, A. E., Evans, W. R., Zaturenskaya, M., & STRONG STAR Training Initiative. (2021). Launching a competency-based training program in evidence-based treatments for PTSD: Supporting veteran-serving mental health providers in Texas. *Community Mental Health Journal, 57,* 910–919.

Dondanville, K. A., Fina, B. A., Straud, C. L., Tyler, H., Jacoby, V., Blount, T. H., Moring, J. C., Blankenship, A. E., & Finley, E. P. (2022). Evaluating a community-based training program for evidence-based treatments for PTSD using the RE-AIM framework. *Psychological Services, 19*(4), 740–750.

Eftekhari, A., Ruzek, J. I., Crowley, J. J., Rosen, C. S., Greenbaum, M. A., & Karlin, B. E. (2013). Effectiveness of national implementation of prolonged exposure therapy in Veterans Affairs care. *JAMA Psychiatry, 70*(9), 949–955.

Ehlers, A., Wild, J., Warnock-Parkes, E., Grey, N., Murray, H., Kerr, A., Rozental, A., Thew, G., Janecka, M., Beierl, E. T., Tsiachristas, A., Perera, R., Andersson, G., & Clark, D. M. (2023). Therapist-assisted online psychological therapies differing in trauma focus for post-traumatic stress disorder (STOP-PTSD): A UK-based, single-blind, randomised controlled trial. *Lancet Psychiatry, 10,* 608–622.

Farmer, C. C., Mitchell, K. S., Parker-Guilbert, K., & Galovski, T. E. (2017). Fidelity to the cognitive processing therapy protocol: Evaluation of critical elements. *Behavior Therapy, 48*(2), 195–206.

Farrell, N. R., Deacon, B. J., Dixon, L. J., & Lickel, J. J. (2013). Theory-based training strategies for modifying practitioner concerns about exposure therapy. *Journal of Anxiety Disorders, 27*(8), 781–787.

Finley, E. P., Garcia, H. A., Ketchum, N. S., McGeary, D. D., McGeary, C. A., Stirman, S. W., & Peterson, A. L. (2015). Utilization of evidence-based psychotherapies in Veterans Affairs posttraumatic stress disorder outpatient clinics. *Psychological Services, 12*(1), 73–82.

Foa, E. B., McLean, C. P., Brown, L. A., Zang, Y., Rosenfield, D., Zandberg, L. J.,... & Peterson, A. L. (2020). The effects of a prolonged exposure workshop with and without consultation on provider and patient outcomes: A randomized implementation trial. *Implementation Science, 15*(1), 1–14.

Forbes, D., Lloyd, D., Nixon, R. D. V., Elliott, P., Varker, T., Perry, D., Bryant, R. A., & Creamer, M. (2012). A multisite randomized controlled effectiveness trial of cognitive processing therapy for military-related posttraumatic stress disorder. *Journal of Anxiety Disorders, 26*(3), 442–452.

Galovski, T. E., Blain, L. M., Mott, J. M., Elwood, L., & Houle, T. (2012). Manualized therapy for PTSD: Flexing the structure of cognitive processing therapy. *Journal of Consulting and Clinical Psychology, 80*(6), 968–981.

Hale, A. C., Sripada, R. K., & Bohnert, K. M. (2018). Past-year treatment utilization among individuals meeting DSM-5 PTSD criteria: Results from a nationally representative sample. *Psychiatric Services, 69*(3), 341–344.

Holder, N., Holliday, R., Williams, R., Mullen, K., & Surís, A. (2018). A preliminary examination of the role of psychotherapist fidelity on outcomes of cognitive processing therapy during an RCT for military sexual trauma-related PTSD. *Cognitive Behaviour Therapy, 47*(1), 76–89.

International Society for Traumatic Stress Studies (ISTSS). (2018). ISTSS PTSD prevention and treatment guidelines: Methodology and recommendations. Retrieved from www.istss.org/getattachment/Treating-Trauma/New-ISTSS-Prevention-and-TreatmentGuidelines/ISTSS_PreventionTreatmentGuidelines_FNL.pdf.aspx

Karlin, B. E., & Cross, G. (2014). From the laboratory to the therapy room: National dissemination and implementation of evidence-based psychotherapies in the US Department of Veterans Affairs Health Care System. *American Psychologist, 69*(1), 19–33.

Karlin, B. E., Ruzek, J. I., Chard, K. M., Eftekhari, A., Monson, C. M., Hembree, E. A.,... & Foa, E. B. (2010). Dissemination of evidence-based psychological treatments for posttraumatic stress disorder in the Veterans Health Administration. *Journal of Traumatic Stress, 23*(6), 663–673.

Kaysen, D., Lindgren, K., Zangana, G. A. S., Murray, L., Bass, J., & Bolton, P. (2013). Adaptation of cognitive processing therapy for treatment of torture victims: Experience in Kurdistan, Iraq. *Psychological Trauma: Theory, Research, Practice, and Policy, 5*(2), 184–192.

Kehle-Forbes, S. M., Ackland, P. E., Spoont, M. R., Meis, L. A., Orazem, R. J., Lyon, A., Valenstein-Mah, H. R., Schnurr, P. P., Zickmund, S. L., Foa, E. B., Chard, K. M., Alpert, E., & Polusny, M. A. (2022). Divergent experiences of US veterans who did and did not complete trauma-focused therapies for PTSD: A national qualitative study of treatment dropout. *Behaviour Research and Therapy, 154*, 104123.

Larsen, S. E., Mackintosh, M. A., La Bash, H., Evans, W. R., Suvak, M. K., Shields, N.,… & Wiltsey Stirman, S. (2022). Temporary PTSD symptom increases among individuals receiving CPT in a hybrid effectiveness-implementation trial: Potential predictors and association with overall symptom change trajectory. *Psychological Trauma: Theory, Research, Practice, and Policy, 14*(5), 853–861.

Lloyd, D., Couineau, A. L., Hawkins, K., Kartal, D., Nixon, R. D., Perry, D., & Forbes, D. (2015). Preliminary outcomes of implementing Cognitive Processing Therapy for post-traumatic stress disorder across a national veterans treatment service. *The Journal of Clinical Psychiatry, 76*(11), 15237.

LoSavio, S. T., Dillon, K. H., Murphy, R. A., Goetz, K., Houston, F., & Resick, P. A. (2019). Using a learning collaborative model to disseminate cognitive processing therapy to community-based agencies. *Behavior Therapy, 50*(1), 36–49.

LoSavio, S. T., Dillon, K. H., Murphy, R. A., & Resick, P. A. (2019). Therapist stuck points during training in cognitive processing therapy: Changes over time and associations with training outcomes. *Professional Psychology: Research and Practice, 50*(4), 255–263.

LoSavio, S. T., Holder, N., Wells, S. Y., & Resick, P. A. (2024). Clinician concerns about cognitive processing therapy: A review of the evidence. *Cognitive and Behavioral Practice, 31*(2), 152–175.

LoSavio, S. T., Worley, C. B., Aajmain, S. T., Rosen, C. S., Wiltsey Stirman, S., & Sloan, D. M. (2023). Effectiveness of written exposure therapy for posttraumatic stress disorder in the Department of Veterans Affairs Healthcare System. *Psychological Trauma: Theory, Research, Practice, and Policy, 15*(5), 748–756.

Maguen, S., Holder, N., Madden, E., Li, Y., Seal, K. H., Neylan, T. C., Lujan, C., Patterson, O. V., DuVall, S. L., & Shiner, B. (2020). Evidence-based psychotherapy trends among posttraumatic stress disorder patients in a national healthcare system, 2001–2014. *Depression and Anxiety, 37*(4), 356–364.

Maguen, S., Madden, E., Holder, N., Li, Y., Seal, K. H., Neylan, T. C., Lujan, C., Patterson, O. V., DuVall, S. L., & Shiner, B. (2023). Effectiveness and comparative effectiveness of evidence-based psychotherapies for posttraumatic stress disorder in clinical practice. *Psychological Medicine, 53*(2), 419–428.

Marques, L., Valentine, S. E., Kaysen, D., Mackintosh, M. A., Dixon De Silva, L. E., Ahles, E. M., Youn, S. J., Shtasel, D. L., Simon, N. M., & Wiltsey-Stirman, S. (2019). Provider fidelity and modifications to cognitive processing therapy in a diverse community health clinic: Associations with clinical change. *Journal of Consulting and Clinical Psychology, 87*(4), 357–369.

McHugh, R. K., & Barlow, D. H. (2010). The dissemination and implementation of evidence-based psychological treatments: A review of current efforts. *American Psychologist, 65*(2), 73–84.

Monson, C. M., Shields, N., Suvak, M. K., Lane, J. E., Shnaider, P., Landy, M. S., Wagner, A. C., Sijercic, I., Masina, T., Wanklyn, S. G., & Stirman, S. W. (2018). A randomized controlled effectiveness trial of training strategies in cognitive processing therapy for posttraumatic stress disorder: Impact on patient outcomes. *Behaviour Research and Therapy, 110*, 31–40.

Murray, L. K., Tol, W., Jordans, M., Zangana, G. S., Amin, A. M., Bolton, P.,…, & Thornicroft, G. (2014). Dissemination and implementation of evidence based, mental health interventions in post conflict, low resource settings. *Intervention (Amstelveen, Netherlands), 12*(Suppl 1), 94–112.

Nadeem, E., Olin, S. S., Hill, L. C., Hoagwood, K. E., & Horwitz, S. M. (2013). Understanding the components of quality improvement collaboratives: A systematic literature review. *The Milbank Quarterly, 91*(2), 354–394.

National Institute for Health and Clinical Practice (NICE). (2018). *Guideline for post-traumatic stress disorder*. London: Author.Pace, B. T., Song, J., Suvak, M. K., Shields, N., Monson, C. M., & Stirman, S. W. (2021). Therapist self-efficacy in delivering cognitive processing therapy in a randomized controlled implementation trial. *Cognitive and Behavioral Practice, 28*(3), 327–335.

Park, J. E., Choi, K. S., Han, Y. R., Kim, J. E., Song, J., Yu, J. C., & Yun, J. A. (2021). An open pilot trial of written exposure therapy for patients with post-traumatic stress disorder in Korea. *Psychiatry Investigation, 18*(8), 728–735.

Phoenix Australia Centre for Posttraumatic Mental Health (Phoenix Australia). (2013). *Australian guidelines for thetreatment of acute stress disorder and posttraumatic stress disorder*. Melbourne: Author.

Powell, B. J., Beidas, R. S., Lewis, C. C., Aarons, G. A., McMillen, J. C., Proctor, E. K., & Mandell, D. S. (2017). Methods to improve the selection and tailoring of implementation strategies. *The Journal of Behavioral Health Services & Research, 44*, 177–194.

Rosner, R., Rimane, E., Frick, U., Gutermann, J., Hagl, M., Renneberg, B., Schreiber, F., Vogel, A., & Steil, R. (2019). Effect of developmentally adapted cognitive processing therapy for youth with symptoms of posttraumatic stress disorder after childhood sexual and physical abuse: A randomized clinical trial. *JAMA Psychiatry, 76*(5), 484–491.

Ruzek, J. I., Eftekhari, A., Rosen, C. S., Crowley, J. J., Kuhn, E., Foa, E. B.,… & Karlin, B. E. (2016). Effects of a comprehensive training program on clinician beliefs about and intention to use prolonged exposure therapy for PTSD. *Psychological Trauma: Theory, Research, Practice, and Policy, 8*(3), 348–355.

Sayer, N. A., Rosen, C. S., Bernardy, N. C., Cook, J. M., Orazem, R. J., Chard, K. M., Mohr, D. C., Kehle-Forbes, S. M, Eftekhari, A., Crowley, J., Ruzek, J. I., Smith, B. N., & Schnurr, P. P. (2017). Context matters: Team and organizational factors associated with reach of evidence-based psychotherapies for PTSD in the Veterans Health Administration. *Administration and Policy in Mental Health and Mental Health Services Research, 44*, 904–918.

Schumm, J. A., Walter, K. H., Bartone, A. S., & Chard, K. M. (2015). Veteran satisfaction and treatment preferences in response to a posttraumatic stress disorder specialty clinic orientation group. *Behaviour Research and Therapy, 69*, 75–82.

Stirman, S. W., Gutner, C. A., Gamarra, J., Suvak, M. K., Vogt, D., Johnson, C., Wachen, J. S., Dondanville, K. A., Yarvis, J. S., Mintz, J., Peterson, A. L., Young-McCaughan, S., Resick, P. A., & STRONG STAR Consortium. (2021). A novel approach to the assessment of fidelity to a cognitive behavioral therapy for PTSD using clinical worksheets: A proof of concept with cognitive processing therapy. *Behavior Therapy, 52*(3), 656–672.

Takagishi, Y., Ito, M., Kanie, A., Morita, N., Makino, M., Katayanagi, A., Sato, T., Imamura, F., Nakajima, S., Oe, Y., Kashimura, M., Kikuchi, A., Narisawa, T., & Horikoshi, M. (2023). Feasibility, acceptability, and preliminary efficacy of cognitive processing therapy in Japanese patients with posttraumatic stress disorder. *Journal of Traumatic Stress, 36*(1), 205–217.

Thompson, R., Simiola, V., Schnurr, P. P., Stirman, S. W., & Cook, J. M. (2018). VA residential treatment providers' use of two evidence-based psychotherapies for PTSD: Global endorsement versus specific components. *Psychological Trauma: Theory, Research, Practice, and Policy, 10*(2), 131–139.

van Minnen, A., Harned, M. S., Zoellner, L., & Mills, K. (2012). Examining potential contraindications for prolonged exposure therapy for PTSD. *European Journal of Psychotraumatology, 3*(1), 18805.

Wachen, J. S., Dondanville, K. A., Evans, W. R., Morris, K., & Cole, A. (2019). Adjusting the timeframe of evidence-based therapies for PTSD-massed treatments. *Current Treatment Options in Psychiatry, 6*, 107–118.

Wilk, J. E., West, J. C., Duffy, F. F., Herrell, R. K., Rae, D. S., & Hoge, C. W. (2013). Use of evidence-based treatment for posttraumatic stress disorder in Army behavioral healthcare. *Psychiatry: Interpersonal and Biological Processes, 76*(4), 336–348.

Worley, C. B., Rosen, C. S., LoSavio, S. T., Aajmain, S. T., Stirman, S. W., & Sloan, D. M. (2023). An examination of individual and organizational theory in a pilot virtual facilitated learning collaborative to implement written exposure therapy. *Psychological Services, 20*(4), 820–830.

Index

Note: Bold page numbers refer to tables.

For Product Safety Concerns and Information please contact our
EU representative GPSR@taylorandfrancis.com Taylor & Francis
Verlag GmbH, Kaufingerstraße 24, 80331 München, Germany